Cognitive Studies in Literature and Performance

This series offers cognitive approaches to understanding perception, emotions, imagination, meaning-making, and the many other activities that constitute both the production and reception of literary texts and embodied performances.

More information about this series at
http://www.palgrave.com/series/14903

Kathryn Banks • Timothy Chesters
Editors

Movement in Renaissance Literature

Exploring Kinesic Intelligence

palgrave
macmillan

Editors
Kathryn Banks
Durham University
Durham, United Kingdom

Timothy Chesters
Cambridge University
Cambridge, United Kingdom

Cognitive Studies in Literature and Performance
ISBN 978-3-319-69199-2 ISBN 978-3-319-69200-5 (eBook)
https://doi.org/10.1007/978-3-319-69200-5

Library of Congress Control Number: 2017963054

Printed on acid-free paper

This Palgrave Macmillan imprint is published by Springer Nature
The registered company is Springer International Publishing AG
The registered company address is: Gewerbestrasse 11, 6330 Cham, Switzerland

Acknowledgements

This book would not have been possible without the generous support of Terence Cave's project, "Thinking with Literature," funded by the Balzan Foundation and St John's College, Oxford. To Terence Cave and those institutions go our warmest thanks. Our interest in kinesic intelligence developed through the exchanges and discussions afforded by the Balzan project (from 2010), on which we both held positions as Research Lecturers. The present volume took shape in a workshop held at Clare College, Cambridge (25–27 September 2014). We are grateful to the participants in the workshop, as well as those in other project events which preceded it.

K.B. and T.C.

Contents

List of Contributors

Kathryn Banks is Associate Professor in French at Durham University. She is the author of *Cosmos and Image in the Renaissance* (2008) and has published essays on Rabelais, sixteenth-century poets, apocalyptic writing, Chrétien de Troyes, and cognitive approaches to literature. She was awarded a Philip Leverhulme Prize in 2013 for research into the specificities of literary thinking.

Guillemette Bolens is Professor of Medieval English Literature and Comparative Literature at the University of Geneva. She is the author of *La Logique du corps articulaire* (2000), *The Style of Gestures: Embodiment and Cognition in Literary Narrative* (2012; French edition 2008), and *L'Humour et le savoir des corps: Don Quichotte, Tristram Shandy et le rire du lecteur* (2016). She has published on embodiment, gestures, and kinesic analysis in Homer, Virgil, *Beowulf*, Chrétien de Troyes, Layamon, the *Gawain* Poet, Chaucer, *Beryn*, Cervantes, Sterne, Proust, Joyce, Chaplin, Keaton, Tati, and Eddie Izzard.

Dominique Brancher is Associate Professor in Humanities (French section) at Basel University. Her research focuses on the interactions between literature and knowledge in the Renaissance (medicine, philosophy, natural philosophy, botany). She is the author of *'Deshonnestes' pudeurs. La fabrique équivoque d'une passion à la Renaissance* and *Quand l'esprit vient aux plantes: botanique sensible et subversion libertine* (both 2015).

Terence Cave is Emeritus Professor of French Literature in the University of Oxford and Emeritus Fellow of St John's College, Oxford. His publications in Renaissance studies include *The Cornucopian Text: Problems of Writing in the French Renaissance* (1979; French translation 1997), *Pré-histoires: textes troublés au seuil de la modernité* (1999), *Pré-histoires II: langues étrangères et troubles économiques au XVIe siècle* (2001), and *How to Read Montaigne* (2007). As the winner of the 2009 Balzan Prize for literature since 1500, he directed a three-year project designed to explore cognitive approaches to literature. His book *Thinking with Literature: Towards a Cognitive Criticism* was published in 2016.

Timothy Chesters is University Lecturer in Sixteenth-Century French Studies and a Fellow of Clare College, Cambridge. He is the author of *Ghost Stories in Late Renaissance France: Walking by Night* (2011). He has also published on Rabelais, Ronsard, Montaigne, nineteenth-century responses to Renaissance writing (with an emphasis on Flaubert), and on cognitive approaches to literature.

Mary T. Crane is the Thomas F. Rattigan Professor of English at Boston College, where she is also director of the Institute for the Liberal Arts. She is the author of *Sayings, Self, and Society in Sixteenth-Century England* (1993); *Shakespeare's Brain: Reading with Cognitive Theory* (2000), and *Losing Touch with Nature: Literature and the New Science in Sixteenth-Century England* (2014).

Ullrich Langer is Alfred Glauser Professor of French at the University of Wisconsin—Madison. His recent publications include *Lyric in the Renaissance: From Petrarch to Montaigne* (2015) and *Penser les formes littéraires du plaisir à la Renaissance* (2009). He is working currently on the "remonstrance" in the French *Ancien Régime* and on movement and the poetry of lamentation in the Renaissance.

Raphael Lyne is a Reader in Renaissance Literature in the Faculty of English, University of Cambridge, and a Fellow of Murray Edwards College. His publications include *Ovid's Changing Worlds: English Metamorphoses, 1567–1632* (2001), *Shakespeare's Late Work* (2007), *Shakespeare, Rhetoric and Cognition* (2011), and *Memory and Intertextuality in Renaissance Literature* (2016). He has also written several articles on cognitive literary theory, and a blog entitled 'What Literature Knows About Your Brain' (http://www.english.cam.ac.uk/research/cogblog/).

Laura Seymour is an Associate Lecturer at Bath Spa University. She completed her PhD on Shakespeare and cognition at the University of London in 2015. She is currently researching enactive cognition in seventeenth-century non-conformist communities thanks to a grant from the Wellcome Trust. Her other book chapters are contained in *The Cognitive Humanities: Embodied Mind in Literature and Culture* (ed. Peter Garratt, 2016) and *Theatre, Performance and Cognition* (ed. Amy Cook and Rhonda Blair, 2016).

Ellen Spolsky is Professor Emerita in the Department of English at Bar-Ilan University in Israel, and a literary theorist with interests centring on the cognitive/epistemological aspects of interpretation and on the embodiment of knowing in language texts and in pictures, as these are manifest in their cultural and historical contexts.

Evelyn Tribble is Professor and Donald Collie Chair of English at the University of Otago, Dunedin, NZ. She is the author of *Margins and Marginality: The Printed Page in Early Modern England* (1993), *Writing Material: Readings from Plato to the Digital Age* (with Anne Trubek, 2003), *Cognitive Ecologies and the History of Remembering* (with Nicholas Keene, 2011), and *Cognition in the Globe: Attention and Memory in Shakespeare's Theatre* (2011). Her book *Early Modern Actors and Shakespeare's Theatre: Thinking with the Body* will be published by Bloomsbury in 2017.

List of Figures

CHAPTER 1

Introduction

Kathryn Banks and Timothy Chesters

> *Let us roll all our strength and all*
> *Our sweetness up into one ball,*
> *And tear our pleasures with rough strife*
> *Through the iron gates of life.*
> —Andrew Marvell, *The Poems of Andrew Marvell*, ed. Nigel Smith (Harlow: Pearson, 2007), 84

When the speaker of Marvell's poem addresses these (almost) closing words to his "coy mistress," exactly what has he communicated? A powerful sense of urgency, certainly, in keeping with the general thrust of the poem as sexual invitation. But just what are readers supposed to see? If we look more closely, this "image" appears a perfect instance of what Christopher Ricks calls Marvell's tendency to transcend the visualizable.[1] The rolled-up ball of strength and sweetness in the first couplet is evidently

We are very grateful to contributors to this volume for their valuable comments on a draft of this Introduction.

K. Banks (✉)
Durham University, Durham, UK

T. Chesters
Clare College, Cambridge, UK

K. Banks, T. Chesters (eds.), *Movement in Renaissance Literature*, Cognitive Studies in Literature and Performance,
https://doi.org/10.1007/978-3-319-69200-5_1

connected to the "tearing through" of the second. But how? Is the ball the thing tearing or the thing torn? "Tear *through* … the iron gates" is unclear too. "With rough strife" could imply the resistance of a closed grill, the pleasures forcibly dragged between its bars. But the gates might equally be open, with a ball-couple tearing along a path through them. Or, perhaps, we might picture the lovers propelling a ball at speed. This faint suggestion is prolonged in the subsequent and final lines of the poem, where we find "one ball" suddenly scaled up to become "our sun" driven along by the poet and his mistress:

> Thus, though we cannot make our sun
> Stand still, yet we will make him run. (84)

And yet all these things the lover's words make visible only obscurely, and possibly not at all.

What does seem certain is that the image engages the body as well as the eye: the action verbs "roll … up" and "tear" prompt a powerful sense of force first gathered then unleashed. Sound and rhythm contribute: in the fricative violence of line 3, and as the pace slows in the spondaic "rough strife" only to rattle through the subsequent line. But acknowledging the centrality of embodiment to the image does not make it any more straightforward. That the poet's mistress might struggle to make global sense of it, for all its embodied immediacy, may not much matter to him. After all immediacy, and not good sense, is precisely what the poet urges: "let's do this violent, constraint-defying thing," he seems to say, "and not worry about the details." The position of the engaged reader or critic, to whom the details do matter, is a little different, however. He or she likewise has no choice but to be struck by the physical shock of Marvell's lines. But this does not mean that the full potential import of the image is experienced with immediacy. What begins as a pre-conscious response is likely to be expanded into a series of more deliberate rehearsals, as we model in more reflective and conscious ways a wide variety of candidate movements to which the verse appears to gesture, such as forcefully pressing through an iron grill or rolling a ball at speed. Thematically speaking, "To His Coy Mistress" pits spontaneity against deliberation, and hopes the first will win. But, cognitively speaking, the poem calls on a mixture of both from careful readers. It calls on what, drawing on work in the cognitive sciences and cognitive humanities, we propose to call their "kinesic intelligence."

Since the latter decades of the twentieth century, the cognitive revolution has transformed disciplines as diverse as linguistics, artificial intelligence, psychology, neuroscience and evolutionary biology. "Cognitive" should not be understood here as restricted to so-called higher-order ratiocinative modes of thinking. As philosopher Ray Jackendoff puts it, "cognition" means "an organism's understanding or grasp of the world and its ability to formulate and execute actions in the world."[2] In other words, the cognitive sciences understand mental processing to be geared towards action, and include within the "cognitive" the non-rational, bodily or emotional. Thus the psychologist Raymond Gibbs warns that "we must not assume cognition to be purely internal, symbolic, computational, and disembodied, but seek out the gross and detailed ways that language and thought are inextricably shaped by embodied action."[3] Indeed, as the philosopher Shaun Gallagher puts it, "the broad argument about the importance of embodiment for understanding cognition has already been made in numerous ways, and there is a growing consensus across a variety of disciplines that this basic fact is inescapable."[4]

We cite Gibbs, Gallagher and Jackendoff to give our readers a sense of the importance of the embodied paradigm in general rather than to align ourselves with any version of it in particular. Conceptions of embodied cognition take diverse forms, and have contributed to diverse cognitive literary research. Particularly influential in the so-called "first wave" of literary cognitivism was work by George Lakoff, Mark Johnson and Mark Turner, which argued that language derived metaphorically from our corporeal and spatially oriented life.[5] More recently, theories of extended mind or distributed cognition (often grouped together as "4E cognition") have come to the fore.[6] Theorists of Extended Mind (EM) understand the cognitive system to include not only the brain but also the body and the world. In common with other second-wave cognitive literary approaches, and our own, Extended Mind presents cognition as a combination of both universal and historical features, emphasizing neural plasticity and the "extension" of human cognition into language and culture. For instance, literary scholars have employed EM to explain how early modern playing companies dealt with the mnemonic burden of performing up to six plays per week, or brought it into dialogue with Renaissance conceptions of cognition and subjectivity as similarly "extended" or "distributed."[7]

Our own approach is grounded in the combination of immediacy and complexity, which we identified in our response to Marvell's "ball." The cognitive sciences focus on mental processing that is too swift to be fully registered in our awareness. Hence Daniel Kahnemann's bestselling *Thinking, Fast and Slow* draws attention to how much of our cognition is extremely rapid. But literary authors and readers, we suggest, engage in a special task, which is to think *both* fast *and* slow. They do this by deploying their "kinesic intelligence."

The term "kinesic intelligence" was first introduced to the critical lexicon by Ellen Spolsky in 1996, borrowed from psychology and neurology.[8] As well as shining a spotlight on our cognitive responses to movement in literature and visual art, Spolsky argued that, especially where art and literature are concerned, embodied knowledge "is not especially privileged in being less ambiguous than other kinds of knowledge."[9] Complexity arose, Spolsky suggested, in the form of conflicts or clashes between bodily knowledge and other forms. Thus Spolsky raised important questions about the degree to which kinesic intelligence was direct or intuitive, and how it related to other modes of knowledge.

Then, armed with insights from more recent scientific work, Guillemette Bolens suggested some new answers to Spolsky's questions.[10] A growing body of research into "motor resonance"—or kinesis—indicates that when we observe the action of another, we access our embodied kinaesthetic memory in order to retrieve a simulation of that action, and so our brains respond in a way similar to when we ourselves execute the movement observed (the phenomenon of so-called "mirror neurons"). Furthermore, motor resonance functions not only when we witness movement but also when we imagine seeing movement, or remember seeing movement, or when we look at visual images of movement, or even when we read a verbal description. Bolens mobilized these insights to argue that "kinesic intelligence in literature is the faculty that enables us to produce and use perceptual simulations in order to understand narrated movements or gestures." *Kinesic* then, is not a synonym for *kinetic*: *kinesis* refers not to movement but rather to the *perception* or understanding of movement.[11]

But literature does not just invite motor simulations in the same way as other visual or linguistic experiences do. Some verbal descriptions are more powerful than others in eliciting sensorimotor responses, and literary texts are often particularly rich in these. For example, Kafka invites sensorimotor responses through strategies of "cognitive realism," as Emily Troscianko has shown.[12] More generally, a broad range of literary texts produce "unpredicted sensorimotor configurations," as Bolens demonstrates.[13] Thus kinesic analysis has as its primary goal "to perceive more keenly and with greater accuracy the potential complexity and subtlety of movements."[14] Complexity, then, is not limited to conflicts between embodied cognition and other kinds, as in Spolsky's earlier work, but emerges in the perception of movements themselves.

Bolens' discussion of complexity also implies that spontaneous pre-reflective simulations might exist on a continuum with the more reflective employment of them. This seems to us a powerful suggestion, potentially rich for literary criticism, and worthy of further exploration. The bodily immediacy of Marvell's images, for example, tips over into—and works together with—a reflective examination of their embodied import. We do not mean to suggest here a definite "tipping point" at which all readers move from immediate pre-reflective response to conscious reflection. Theories of embodied cognition precisely indicate that so-called "higher order" cognitive modes are grounded in bodily ones, so it seems more plausible to speak, as Terence Cave has done, of a gradient between the pre-reflective and the reflective.[15] Nor do we wish to suggest that immediate bodily responses pre-determine the precise meanings we ascribe to texts. However, it seems to us that sense-making and embodied responses should not be considered in isolation from each other but might work together within some kind of feedback loop. Immediate responses might prompt us to reflect at more length on movements such as tearing through a grille and rolling a ball. At the same time, reflecting on a passage might affect its impact on our body on a subsequent reading. But precisely how embodied cognition interacts with conscious reflection remains an open question. The essays in this book are a series of soundings in this combination of thinking fast and slow, in how literature can make kinesis shade into kinesic intelligence.

Claiming an integral role for body, movement and action in the interpretation of literary minds is not new. In the middle of the last century Maurice Merleau-Ponty's concept of "motor intentionality" informed the work of the so-called Geneva-School critics—notably Jean Rousset, Jean-Pierre Richard and Jean Starobinski. This "criticism of consciousness" took for granted Merleau-Ponty's assumption that "my body is my point of view on the world," that my grip on others' intentional states *just is* an attunement to the movements, gestures, and postures of their body.[16] Starobinski's *Montaigne in Motion*, a model of this approach, remains a landmark of French Renaissance studies; and one might also consider Bolens, a more recent Geneva critic, as belonging broadly in this tradition while extending it in new directions.[17] Merleau-Ponty's insights have recently gained new traction in the work of Alva Noë and Shaun Gallagher, whose phenomenologically inflected cognitive philosophy has found an enthusiastic following among literary scholars with an interest in social cognition and empathy. Gallagher's phenomenology has led him to be cautious of the motor resonance system, whose "subpersonal" routines are not present to our awareness; others have regarded the echoic traces it produces as the neural correlate of what Merleau-Ponty termed *entrelacs*—the chiasmic intertwining of self, other and world.

The concept of "kinesic intelligence," as applied to literary texts, both builds on this work and moves beyond it. A key assumption of phenomenological criticism is that the intentions of others are always already immanent to us in experience, that their bodies are easily legible to us. We claim that while this may ring true for many of our everyday interactions, the "unpredicted sensorimotor configurations" described by Bolens as characteristic of literature pose a special kind of problem. One feature not unique to literary communication, but certainly amplified in it, is the degree to which it requires a heightened attunement to kinesic effects. These can feel overpoweringly immediate ("Pray you undo this button,") and so accessible to a more unreflective mode of kinesic intelligence.[18] But often this immediacy combines with degrees of kinesic opacity and complexity, like those of Marvell's "ball." Such opacity calls for a more reflective response—even the exercise of *criticism*.

A preoccupation with opaque or complex movement also distinguishes our approach from some of the work being done under the banner of cognitive linguistics. For Lakoff, Johnson and Turner, our conceptual architecture is so comprehensively grounded in embodiment that even the most abstruse linguistic formulations reflect a limited set of metaphor kernels, or "metaphors we live by." On this view the closing lines of Marvell's "To His Coy Mistress" might be analysed as a blend of LOVE-IS-A-FORCE and LIFE-IS-A-JOURNEY, for example. While this undoubtedly imparts something about the general conceptual grounding of Marvell's verses, the more interesting challenge, to our minds, is to capture the specific force of the images as they are developed in these particular lines. This would include accounting for the fact that, lacking the simplicity of the Lakoffian X-is-Y structure, the spatio-visual content of Marvell's metaphors remains so tricky to pin down. Such messiness is not at all atypical of literary utterances; rather than tidy it away, reading with kinesic intelligence means accepting and analysing cognitive effort, frustration, even failure.[19]

Moreover, insofar as conceptual metaphor approaches focus on the level of the "underlying" metaphor, they pay scant attention to history and context. Therefore, like other cognitive literary studies, which foreground apparently universal aspects of cognition, some conceptual metaphor studies draw accusations of a fundamental incompatibility between the cognitive sciences and literary studies. However, these disciplines have much to learn from each other precisely because "literary utterances reflect in especially rich ways the situatedness of cognition itself," as Terence Cave puts it.[20] Bolens demonstrates the "situatedness" of specifically kinesic intelligence with reference to the very particular nineteenth-century world of Jane Austen's *Pride and Prejudice*. Mr Darcy arrives back at Pemberley where, to his great astonishment, he finds Elizabeth Bennett. The narrator states: "He absolutely started, and for a moment seemed immoveable from surprise." Though Austen supplies the word "surprise" here, it is hard to see how this word could ever fix—semanticize—the complex tug of contradictory kineses prompted by the sentence as a whole. What kind of intentionality can we attribute to an *absolute starting*—that is, a motion both fully formed and incipient, vigorous and withheld at one and the same time? Bolens shows that the only way to proceed here is to *contextualize* Darcy's movement, both within that character's overall kinesic style, and within the social conventions of expression and restraint that governed Austen's world.[21] Movement arises within a cognitive ecology, and history, context and style are central to the complex cognitive ecologies of literary texts.

But how might an approach grounded in kinesic intelligence be pertinent to the Renaissance in particular? The image on the cover of this book points to one answer. This image—a fresco from the wall of Cosimo de' Medici's Palazzo Vecchio in Florence—is, if nothing else, one of bodies in movement. It reworks one version of the well-known iconography of the popular Renaissance proverb "Festina lente," variously a butterfly atop a crab, a tortoise with sail as here, or Aldus Manutius's dolphin-encircled anchor. The "festina lente"—employed to indicate, among other things, the governor's combination of incisiveness and prudence—bore the authority of *doxa*, the wisdom of the ages. But how did it earn this status? What special quality ensured its success? Erasmus, who discourses at length on the motto in his *Adages,* finds in the proverb a "charming riddle," owing its "gem-like grace" to its "apt and absolute brevity" and its applicability to "every activity of life." But Cosimo's fresco hints at another possible reason for the proverb's success.

The fresco heeds "festina lente" not only as an ethical command but also as a complex injunction to bodies called upon to perform an impossible movement. The five *putti* introduced into the usually static juxtaposition of tortoise and sail give rise to a combination of pulling, pushing and prompting; the tautness of ropes and tendons set against the billowing sail invite viewers to feel the contrary pressure of upward flight and countervailing gravity. The fresco thus foregrounds a contradiction at the heart of the *festina lente*, present in the words of the proverb but dulled by its familiarity: the impossibility of the imperative addressed to a body with an acute sense of its inability to "hasten slowly." In other words, the fresco offers an example of Renaissance culture revivifying the embodied. It suggests that Renaissance humanism was not just about renewing linguistic forms, where language is conceived in a non-material sense, or renewing ethics, conceived as *doxa* frozen in language. Instead, what was reborn in the Renaissance was, in part, a critical sense of the capacities and complexities of bodily movement. Like Cosimo's fresco, we suggest, literary texts engage anew with kinesic intelligence.

A striking instance of this is provided by Rabelais who, as Kathryn Banks shows, stimulates kinesic intelligence by infusing the proverbial with new life. Rabelais's oft-noted shifts between the "metaphorical" and the "literal"—and, more broadly, between the more embodied or the more abstract—invite corresponding switches in readers' cognitive responses; those responses were further shaped by humanism and its notion of a "seamless web" of language. In Scève's poetry, too, the linguistic ingenuity characteristic of Renaissance humanism called for acute sensorimotor attunement from its readers, as Timothy Chesters demonstrates. Chesters draws attention to the denominal verbs coined by Scève, arguing that readers understand these by inferring complex movements from minimal verbal cues. But language mediates sensorimotor responses through syntax as well as lexis, as Terence Cave shows in his analysis of chiasmus as a kinesic figure in Montaigne's essays and Scève's poetry. Ullrich Langer examines gestures that are archetypal in the Western tradition—Orpheus turning back to look at his wife, Eurydice, and Eurydice reaching out to her husband. Lyric by Petrarch and subsequent French poets reimagines these gestures, thereby showing that the physical movements underlying figurative ones can appeal powerfully to kinesic intelligence, and, in this case, with extensive implications for ethics.

Kinesic intelligence can also be embodied in the theatre. The "skill" of the early modern actor shaped his body, as Evelyn Tribble demonstrates with reference to "age transvestism" in Shakespeare and John Marston. Raphael Lyne shows how Shakespearean actors who "play dead" engage the kinesic intelligence of their audience through vital signs—senses of weight, warmth, pulse, breath and muscular tension—which explore what it feels like to be alive. In Laura Seymour's study of "exchanging hands" in *Titus Andronicus*, actions embodied on stage bear a complex relation to figurative actions. Imagery is also Mary Crane's focus, specifically the metaphorical choking, suffocation and balked movement of *Macbeth*.

Finally, kinesic intelligence casts new light on established critical preoccupations concerning the body—gender, sexuality and violence. How does gender inflect kinesic response? Dominique Brancher investigates this by examining movement inflicted on somebody who defies gender categories, as presented in Jacques Duval's 1612 *Traité des hermaphrodits*. And violence takes centre stage in Guillemette Bolens' analysis of the crucifix deployed as weapon in Folengo and Rabelais, which Bolens assesses in relation to Renaissance developments in artillery.

Thus this volume explores kinesic intelligence at work across a rich array of Renaissance experience. Readers are invited to trace their own paths through an assortment of Renaissance movements: the order of chapters in *Movement in Renaissance Literature* is not intended to mirror every reader's trajectory. We ask of our readers only that they both register the embodied responses described here and also engage with them critically—that is, that they think both fast and slow.

Notes

1. *The Force of Poetry* (Oxford: Oxford University Press, 1984), 41.
2. *Language, Consciousness, Culture: Essays on Mental Structure* (Cambridge, MA: MIT Press, 2007), 3.
3. *Embodiment and Cognitive Science* (Cambridge: Cambridge University Press), 9.
4. *How The Body Shapes the Mind* (Oxford: Oxford University Press, 2005), 1.
5. For a recent example of an approach to renaissance literature inspired by cognitive linguistics, see Amy Cook, *Shakespearean Neuroplay: Reinvigorating the Study of Dramatic Texts and Performance Through Cognitive Science* (New York: Palgrave Macmillan, 2010).
6. 4E is a mnemonic referring to embodied, embedded, enactive and extended accounts of cognition—overlapping theories of cognition as extended across brain, body and world.
7. Evelyn Tribble, *Cognition in the Globe: Attention and Memory in Shakespeare's Theatre* (New York: Palgrave Macmillan, 2011). Miranda Anderson, *The Renaissance Extended Mind* (New York: Palgrave Macmillan, 2015). See also Evelyn Tribble and Nicholas Keene, *Cognitive Ecologies and the History of*

Remembering: Religion, Education and Memory in Early Modern England (Basingstoke: Palgrave Macmillan, 2011); Lina Perkins Wilder, *Shakespeare's Memory Theatre: Recollection, Properties, and Character* (Cambridge: Cambridge University Press, 2010).

8. "Elaborated Knowledge: Reading Kinesis in Pictures," *Poetics Today* 17 (1996): 157–80. Spolsky's *Satisfying Skepticism: Embodied Knowledge in the Early Modern World* (Aldershot: Ashgate, 2001) brings the notion of a "sympathetic kinaesthetic sense" to bear on literature as well as art. The concept of kinesic intelligence was deployed by Oliver Sacks, and by Howard Gardner in his account of multiple intelligences.
9. "Elaborated Knowledge," 168.
10. *Le Style des gestes: Corporéité et kinésie dans le récit littéraire* (Lausanne: BHMS, 2008). English version: *The Style of Gestures: Embodiment and Cognition in Literary Narrative* (Baltimore: The Johns Hopkins University Press, 2012).
11. Why do we refer to both the "kinaesthetic" and the "kinesic" here? "Kinaesthesis" means our sense or perception of our bodies moving (http://www.oed.com/view/Entry/103437?redirectedFrom=kinaesthetic#eid40177097). So kinaesthetic memory or kinaesthetic knowledge denote our memory or knowledge of how it feels to perform a movement or hold a bodily posture. By contrast, by "kinesis" we mean our *perception* and simulation of the movement of other humans or animals or things, including as it is portrayed on the stage or in language. And "kinesic intelligence," as we shall explain more fully, refers to our capacity to discern and to interpret bodily movements and postures, and operates on a continuum from the pre-reflective to the reflective. "Kinetic" has, of course, a more general sense, referring simply to any kind of motion.
12. *Kafka's Cognitive Realism* (New York: Routledge, 2014).
13. *Style of Gestures*, 17.
14. *Style of Gestures*, 9.
15. *Thinking with Literature: Towards a Cognitive Criticism* (Oxford: Oxford University Press, 2016), 21–4, 40–2.
16. Merleau-Ponty, *Phenomenology of Perception*, trans. Colin Smith (London: Routledge, 2002), 81. Sarah Lawall, *Critics of Consciousness: The Existential Structures of Literature* (Cambridge, MA: Harvard University Press, 1968).
17. Starobinski, *Montaigne in Motion*, trans. Arthur Goldhammer (Chicago: University of Chicago Press, 1985).
18. On vivid imagery and the special role played by motion, see G. Gabrielle Starr, *Feeling Beauty: The Neuroscience of Aesthetic Experience* (Cambridge, MA: MIT Press, 2015), 81–100; id, "Theorizing Imagery, Aesthetics, and Doubly Directed States," in *The Oxford Handbook of Cognitive Literary*

Studies, ed. Lisa Zunshine (New York: Oxford University Press, 2015), 246–68; Elaine Scarry, *Dreaming by the Book* (New York: Farrar, Strauss and Giroux, 1999).
19. On literature and failures of cognition, see Ellen Spolsky, *The Contracts of Fiction: Cognition, Culture, Community* (New York: Oxford University Press, 2015), 130–154; and Spolsky, "An Embodied View of Misunderstanding in *Macbeth*," *Poetics Today* 2011 (32): 489–520.
20. Terence Cave, "Situated Cognition: The Literary Archive," in *Poetics Today* 38 (2017): 235–53. See also Mark J. Bruhn and Donald R. Wehrs, eds, *Cognition, Literature, and History* (New York: Routledge, 2014).
21. Bolens, *Style of Gestures*, 28–33.

Bibliography

Anderson, Miranda. *The Renaissance Extended Mind*. New York: Palgrave Macmillan, 2015.

Bolens, Guillemette. *Le Style des gestes: Corporéité et kinésie dans le récit littéraire*. Lausanne: BHMS, 2008.

———. *The Style of Gestures: Embodiment and Cognition in Literary Narrative*. Baltimore: The Johns Hopkins University Press, 2012.

Bruhn, Mark J., and Donald R. Wehrs, eds. *Cognition, Literature, and History*. New York: Routledge, 2014.

Cave, Terence. *Thinking with Literature: Towards a Cognitive Criticism*. Oxford: Oxford University Press, 2016.

———. Situated Cognition: The Literary Archive. *Poetics Today* 38 (2017): 235–53.

Cook, Amy. *Shakespearean Neuroplay: Reinvigorating the Study of Dramatic Texts and Performance Through Cognitive Science*. New York: Palgrave Macmillan, 2010.

Gallagher, Shaun. *How the Body Shapes the Mind*. Oxford: Oxford University Press, 2005.

Gibbs, Raymond. *Embodiment and Cognitive Science*. Cambridge: Cambridge University Press, 2005.

Jackendoff, Ray. *Language, Consciousness, Culture: Essays on Mental Structure*. Cambridge, MA: MIT Press, 2007.

Lawall, Sarah. *Critics of Consciousness: The Existential Structures of Literature*. Cambridge, MA: Harvard University Press, 1968.

Marvell, Andrew. *The Poems of Andrew Marvell*. Edited by Nigel Smith. Harlow: Pearson, 2007.

Merleau-Ponty, Maurice. *Phenomenology of Perception*. Translated by Colin Smith. London: Routledge, 2002.

Ricks, Christopher. *The Force of Poetry*. Oxford: Oxford University Press, 1984.

Scarry, Elaine. *Dreaming by the Book*. New York: Farrar, Strauss and Giroux, 1999.
Spolsky, Ellen. Elaborated Knowledge: Reading Kinesis in Pictures. *Poetics Today* 17 (1996): 157–80.
———. *Satisfying Skepticism: Embodied Knowledge in the Early Modern World*. Aldershot: Ashgate, 2001.
———. An Embodied View of Misunderstanding in *Macbeth*. *Poetics Today* 32 (2011): 489–520.
———. *The Contracts of Fiction: Cognition, Culture, Community*. New York: Oxford University Press, 2015.
Starobinski, Jean. *Montaigne in Motion*. Translated by Arthur Goldhammer. Chicago: University of Chicago Press, 1985.
Starr, G. Gabrielle. *Feeling Beauty: The Neuroscience of Aesthetic Experience*. Cambridge, MA: MIT Press, 2015a.
———. Theorizing Imagery, Aesthetics, and Doubly Directed States. In *The Oxford Handbook of Cognitive Literary Studies*, edited by Lisa Zunshine, 246–68. New York: Oxford University Press, 2015b.
Tribble, Evelyn. *Cognition in the Globe: Attention and Memory in Shakespeare's Theatre*. New York: Palgrave Macmillan, 2011.
Tribble, Evelyn, and Nicholas Keene. *Cognitive Ecologies and the History of Remembering: Religion, Education and Memory in Early Modern England*. Basingstoke: Palgrave Macmillan, 2011.
Troscianko, Emily. *Kafka's Cognitive Realism*. New York: Routledge, 2014.
Wilder, Lina Perkins. *Shakespeare's Memory Theatre: Recollection, Properties, and Character*. Cambridge: Cambridge University Press, 2010.

CHAPTER 2

Chiastic Cognition: Kinesic Intelligence Between the Reflective and the Pre-reflective in Montaigne and Scève

Terence Cave

The value of the notions of kinesis and kinesic intelligence is that they offer a particularly focused variant of so-called second-generation cognitive studies. They address the problem of embodied mind in a way that is flexible, avoiding the ontological extravagance of some philosophical approaches, while making salient the fine details of particular modes of mind–body interaction. For these reasons, they are especially well suited to literary analysis in a cognitive perspective, as well as to studies in the visual arts, film and related media: it is no accident that Guillemette Bolens uses Chardin's painting of the boy with a top as a frontispiece for *Le Style des gestes* and speaks of the body in action in case-studies of Tati, Chaplin and Keaton.[1]

These terms also have the advantage that they are flexible: defining them is not a question of setting boundaries and insisting on rigorous exclusions. A working definition of kinesis, valid for my present purposes but open to eventual modification, might run as follows: "the mutual reading of bodily movement and gesture, grounded in motor resonance." What is meant by "motor resonance" is that the observer of a salient physical action, gesture or bodily posture will experience an echoic trace of that action in their own

T. Cave (✉)
St John's College, Oxford, UK

K. Banks, T. Chesters (eds.), *Movement in Renaissance Literature*,
Cognitive Studies in Literature and Performance,
https://doi.org/10.1007/978-3-319-69200-5_2

body via the automatic activation of their motor neurons. The word "observer" here evokes a typical scene: I see a student in an examination hall, biting his nails over a difficult question, and feel an uncomfortable and mildly distressing echo of the tension in his hands, his face, his whole posture. The feeling is automatic, unreflective. Crucially for present purposes, however, research in this area has widely shown that physical presence is not essential. An appropriate description of the same phenomenon can trigger the same effects. Language—not only lexical items, but also syntactical markers—is saturated with bodily inputs, not least because it is normally acquired situationally; it has strong sensorimotor connections. The nail-biting I have described is already producing its resonance in my body and perhaps in yours, too, if you allow it to become salient for you. In other words, language (whether oral or written) can successfully mediate motor resonance, even enhance it, while inserting it into the whole network of cultural and conceptual resources that individual humans have at their disposal. It is important to emphasize that we are not talking here about top-down symbolic representation of the body; this is bottom-up reading, which brings to the reflective surface traces of the reader's pre-reflective sensorimotor response. We should also note here already that, in order for this to happen, a high degree of kinesic intelligence must be pre-supposed on the side of the writer: kinesis is always at least potentially a reciprocal activity.

The first part of this paper will consist of a close kinesic reading of the opening page of Montaigne's chapter "De l'institution des enfans" (*Essais* I.26), designed to establish that "bottom-up" mode.[2] I shall then look at some instances of chiasmus as a cognitive (and more specifically kinesic) figure, both in Montaigne's *Essais* and in one of the *dizains* from Maurice Scève's *Délie*. This development will in turn lead to some remarks on the question of the primacy or otherwise of cultural and historical specificity in what is essentially a cognitive methodology, and on the relation between the reflective and the pre-reflective in the reading process, taken here to include what is presumed to be the writer's degree of awareness of such effects.

The Movement of Thought: Montaigne's Gestural Style

Here is Montaigne's initial sketch, at the opening of "De l'institution des enfans," of his response to formal education, no doubt with nail-biting memories of his youth:

> [E]n somme, je sçay qu'il y a une Medecine, une Jurisprudence, quatre parties en la Mathematique, et grossierement ce à quoy elles visent. Mais, d'y enfoncer plus avant, de m'estre rongé les ongles à l'estude d'Aristote, ou opiniastré après quelque science, je ne l'ay jamais faict.[3]

> [Briefly put, I know that there's something called Medicine, and Jurisprudence, and four types of Mathematics, and very roughly what they're supposed to be for. But to delve more deeply into them, to have chewed my nails to the quick over the study of Aristotle, or to go in dogged pursuit of some area of knowledge, I've never done that.]

The second sentence of this passage is full of friction, resistance, tension. The kinesic verb "enfoncer" triggers a muscular sense of pushing against an obstacle, breaking through a resistant surface; nail-biting delivers a variant of that response,[4] coupled with a tense position of the hand, arm and face; "opiniastré" echoes the same tension, a mental stance rooted in a bodily one (obstinacy is immediately visible in the body and face). These tensions are negated ("Je ne l'ay jamais faict"), but after the event, so that the sentence reads like an instance of *praeteritio*. The motor resonance is evoked before it is cancelled. More generally, however, the tension is framed by the informal, everyday syntax and the (self)-irony: the whole sequence is neatly balanced between tension and relaxation.

In the ensuing sentences, the kinesic mode—bodily posture, attitude, expressive tonus[5] reified in language—shifts between those two poles, which, as Ellen Spolsky has pointed out, are fundamental to our sensorimotor understanding of human movement and agency.[6] First there is a palpable relaxation, a sigh of relief, as we shift to the subjects Montaigne professes to prefer:

> L'Histoire, c'est plus mon gibier, ou la poësie, que j'ayme d'une particuliere inclination.

> [History is more my cup of tea, or poetry, for which I have a special fondness.]

The implicatures[7] of "gibier" (literally "quarry") might include something better than nails to chew on; but hunting, unlike sitting indoors poring over Aristotle, is also one of the outdoor pursuits of the gentry. Such implicatures harmonize with the tension-releasing diction, phrased in the mode of oral speech (the subject thrown out first, then confirmed with a demonstrative pronoun). What is immediately evident here is that the barely detectable kinesic effect of "gibier" (implying a readiness for pursuit, the open air) is rapidly overtaken by the gestural rhythm of the sentence. That rhythm includes the scalar expression "plus": it gently guides the reader towards an opening possibility, a more comfortable path. By the time we arrive at "ou," the body is already relaxed, at ease with itself.

So now let us focus for a moment on that little word. As used here, "ou" is not a logical operator; like the scalar "plus," it is a procedural expression, in other words, a linguistic feature that guides the reader's (or interlocutor's) interpretation of the propositional content of the utterance.[8] It communicates the speaker's attitude and even his posture: try reading Montaigne's sentence aloud and you'll find yourself *performing* the permissive gesture, the opening to new possibilities, which it implies. In other words, this tiny conjunction has a kinesic function: it is easy to assume that kinesis is delivered mainly by verbs and adverbs, but in fact any element of language, including the movement of a sentence, can give rise to kinesic effects. At the same time, the procedural "ou" is also the marker of an improvisational shift of topic or interest. Montaigne is thinking on the wing.[9] The second of the two items proposed becomes the subject of the next sentence; history is left behind for now:

> Car, comme disoit Cleantes, tout ainsi que la voix, contrainte dans l'étroit canal d'une trompette, sort plus aiguë et plus forte, ainsi me semble il que la sentence, pressée aux pieds nombreux de la poësie, s'eslance bien plus brusquement et me fiert d'une plus vive secousse.
>
> [For, as Cleanthes used to say, just as the voice, when forced through the narrow passage of a trumpet, sounds sharper and louder when it comes out, so too, it seems to me, a thought, when constrained by the rhythmic feet of poetry, comes across more powerfully and strikes me a livelier blow.]

What is immediately remarkable about that sentence is its tightly constrained energy, its *tension*. The energy is embodied both in its syntax and rhythm, and in the figurative equivalence it proposes: a formal and highly symmetrical simile, the phrases taut but pliably balanced, definitely not the kind of sentence you improvise.

The key conceptual item in this equivalence is the word "sentence" (thought): what is demonstrated here is the way in which the acoustic kinesis of poetry delivers a conceptual payload that is bound to its embodied form. Its effect becomes palpable in the kinesic final phrase "me fiert d'une plus vive secousse." The writer's body here is in passive mode, receiving a sharp blow, "me fiert": the slightly anachronistic verb carries implicatures of epic and romance battles. Phenomenally, the blow is registered as a shock: the body is *shaken* by the impact. The shock or impact of poetry is palpable throughout the *Essais*, and we shall return to it later. But here Montaigne rebounds from it to another level, the relaxed level of his own discourse:

> Quant aux facultez naturelles qui sont en moy, dequoy c'est icy l'essay, je les sens flechir sous la charge.
>
> [As for my own natural faculties, which I'm putting to the test here, I feel them giving way under that pressure.]

From "me fiert" to "flechir," the tension shifts markedly. "I feel them giving way" makes the phenomenal perspective even more salient, but the shock has been replaced by an accommodating response of the body to pressure: "flechir" resonates with an *evasive* movement, designed to cushion the impact, *reduce* the shock. The rebound, the relaxation of tension, also (automatically, without reflection) colours the conceptual payload: while the body is foregrounded here, the nominal subject is the "mind," the cognitive faculties. The kinesic is bound to the conceptual and vice versa.

From the unspecified particular *sententia* of the poetry sentence via the collective designation of cognitive faculties located *within* the writer ("[les] facultez naturelles qui sont en moy"), we come then to a third formulation of the conceptual payload, articulated by a further set of kinesic gestures:

> Mes conceptions et mon jugement ne marche qu'à tastons, chancelant, bronchant et chopant ; et, quand je suis allé le plus avant que je puis, si ne me suis-je aucunement satisfaict; je voy encore du païs au delà, mais d'une veuë trouble et en nuage, que je ne puis desmeler.
>
> [My conceptions and my judgement can only grope their way forward, staggering, stumbling and tripping; and when I have gone as far as I am able, I am still in no way satisfied; I can see further terrain in the distance, but with a murky, cloudy vision which I'm unable to resolve.]

Let us begin here with the triad "chancelant, bronchant et chopant." This is a classic kinesic sequence of quasi-synonymous verbs. They calibrate similar but significantly different kinds of movement. Guillemette Bolens points out that English is especially rich in these, but Montaigne's sixteenth-century French was rich in them too, and no one knew better how to select them than he did: that is precisely what is meant by kinesic intelligence as a faculty of the writer. It is no doubt worth mentioning that, although kinesic effect is not dependent on devices such as onomatopoeia, sound-values do count in this domain (think of the English cluster slide-slither-slip-skid), and the swishing, shifting "ch" sound is a salient, audible feature of the overall kinesic effect. The articulated voice is not just a vehicle of motor resonance, but is itself a kinesic stimulus.

Secondly: the walking body that becomes palpable in this sentence has a habitus, a characteristic gait: it can *only* walk gropingly ("ne marche qu'*à tastons*"). The gait is constitutionally uncertain, unpredictable, improvised. At the same time, this uncertain gait is given a special kinesic turn by the etymology of "taster": to touch, to feel, to try out by touching; "à tastons" is a haptic expression, as indeed were the verbs of staggering, tripping and stumbling. As Hugo Friedrich pointed out long ago, "taster" is semantically connected with "essayer," so the kinesic thread that connects this and the previous sentence becomes more complex, carries more implicatures, as it proceeds.

Thirdly: the subject "mes conceptions et mon jugement" echoes the "facultez naturelles" of the previous sentence. It is an abstract subject, delivering the conceptual payload; and it is also a *plural* subject for a *singular* verb ("marche"). You might say that a singular body (which does the "walking") unifies the writer's collective "mental faculties." We are talking here, then, about a cognitive apparatus that is embodied from the outset; the conceptual is yet again folded into the kinesic, delivered kinesically. Is this a metaphor? Well, in a sense, yes. But I want to insist here that this isn't just a question of Montaigne's preference for metaphor, as if metaphor were purely instrumental and operated at a less ontologically privileged level. These metaphors are *literal*, in the sense that the thinking body isn't a fiction, an ad hoc invention. There is nothing but a body that does the thinking. There is no purely conceptual level of meaning.[10]

***

It may be helpful here to review what has happened to the thread of argument that began with "L'histoire, c'est plus mon gibier, ou ...." From history (not further discussed) it takes us provisionally to poetry as a kinesic vector of thought (one sentence). So far, so good. Poetry delivers a certain kind of cognitive shock, registered in first-person mode ("*me* fiert"). The shock is prolonged in the kinesic gesture of yielding to pressure, articulated as a *feeling* ("je les sens fleschir sous la charge"). But is this still the pressure of poetic thought and form? Grammatically, that is what must be inferred. But the first person has by now become the whole ground of cognitive experience ("Quant aux facultez naturelles qui sont en moy"), and Montaigne speaks of his own writing, "dequoy c'est icy l'essay." In that light, one has to revise one's inference. Montaigne can't do poetry, or indeed formal prose of the kind the poetry sentence has exemplified; he can only do essays, with their suite of kinesic articulations. And he is no longer speaking of the occasional experience of reading poetry; he is speaking of a whole way of thinking. Poetry is a mode of thought Montaigne admires (and integrates into his text) but cannot emulate; the "essaying" mode offers instead its slacker, more accommodating gestures, made salient by the rebound effect. And so we grope our way forward again towards an even longer, less symmetrical sentence, this time about thinking with the Ancients, and specifically with Plutarch on the imagination.[11] The coherence and directedness of the thread seems almost accidental.

Chiasmus as Kinesis

The movement of the passage we have so far been looking at shifts, then, between poetry and the mode of the "essay" on the one hand, between the kinesic and the conceptual on the other. As it moves, it binds these topics, fusing them in a single sustained reflection on the way thought can be articulated beyond the constraints of Aristotelian or mathematical logic, or of thought as officially encoded knowledge. A few years later, Montaigne returns to this nexus in "Sur des vers de Virgile" (*Essais*, III.5) via the lines of erotic Latin verse referred to in the title, together with a parallel passage from Lucretius. As in I.26, these extraordinary (and richly kinesic) passages become a paradigm of poetry as a mode of thought that ostensibly puts to shame the feeble vernacular writing of Montaigne's own day; but here again, as in I.26, the movement of contrast is overlaid by the palpable energies of Montaigne's own kinesic style as he meditates on what it is that makes such writing come uniquely alive. As I show elsewhere,[12] the key move is the addition of two words to a tiny fragment from Juvenal quoted immediately after the eponymous lines from Virgil: "*Et versus* digitos habet" ("[A line of poetry too] has fingers") (849). Montaigne reads the kinesis of Virgil's poetry as haptic; also, one might note, as communicative, reaching out, not to grope in this case, but to caress the reader. These stroking fingers, heavily laden with erotic implicatures, create the kinesic impetus for a complex development that stretches across many pages of the chapter.

A critical point in that development is reached with a striking chiasmus. It is located just after the commentary on the parallel erotic passage from Lucretius, and it expresses the reciprocal relation between poetic language and thought:

> Quand je voy ces braves formes de s'expliquer, si vifves, si profondes, je ne dicts pas que c'est bien dire, je dicts que c'est bien penser. C'est la gaillardise de l'imagination qui esleve et enfle les parolles. [C] "*Pectus est quod disertum facit*" [B] Nos gens appellent jugement, langage; et beaux mots, les plaines conceptions. (873)
>
> [When I see those bold forms of communication,[13] so alive, so profound, I don't say "That's well said," I say "That's well thought." It is the joyful vigour of the imagination that raises and swells the words. [C] '*It is intuition that makes the speaker eloquent.*' [B] People nowadays call judgement "language"; and "fine words," full conceptions.[14]]

The claim that poetic language is a way of thinking could hardly be put more explicitly or more strongly. Here, once again, are the "conceptions" and the "jugement" of I.26, together with the poetic *sentence* that delivers its kinesic payload as a shock or blow. This time, however, thought takes on the colour of "imagination," a word Montaigne often uses in the broadened sense of something like an embodied concept. Embodied enough, clearly, to be explicitly erotic, even sexual: "c'est la gaillardise de l'imagination qui esleve et enfle les paroles" takes its upwardly mobile kinesic cues from sexual arousal.[15] Yet the crossing-over or exchange required to achieve authentic embodiment works in exactly the same way as in I.26. The language enacts the sexual body, which becomes identified reciprocally with thought, "les plaines conceptions."

So now to the cross-over step performed by the chiasmus. A word is needed first, perhaps, to raise a question about how Montaigne means us to read it. Who are "Nos gens"? Are they his French contemporaries whose vernacular lacks the sinews of classical Latin? Is he being ironic? The sense would then be that we/they debase "jugement" and "les plaines conceptions" by identifying them as mere rhetoric. I have gestured towards that possible sense by translating "Nos gens" as "People nowadays," a version that is in accord with a number of modern commentaries and translations. But "nos gens" could also mean "our servants," "the people who work for us": ordinary people who, although uneducated, have a firm sense of realities. Such a meaning is present on the next page of this same chapter when Montaigne says that his page-boy can make love (in the older sense of that expression) and understand it; if you read Leone Ebreo and Marsilio Ficino to him, he will be none the wiser (874). The context here is different, but I think it is possible that Montaigne is pointing to a speech habit of ordinary people, who identify high-flying thought, without irony, as "fine words."

Whoever "nos gens" may be, and however ironic the phrase, the chiasmus works in the same way. It identifies thought (*imagination*) with language, and more specifically the heightened language of poetry. The trumpet blast of I.26 and the reaching fingers of III.5 are cognitive affordances fashioned by remarkably talented wordsmiths and available to anyone with the kinesic intelligence to read them. Montaigne's prose may give way under the pressure, but it has resources of its own. It is capable, for example, of fashioning an affordance (the chiasmus) that displays the reciprocal duality of poetry-as-thought, like the duck that is also, when inverted, a rabbit.

One way of defining chiasmus is to think of it as a sequential mode of binding or merging. You take one step forward, then reverse the movement: that *turn* locks the two elements together, like a turn of the wrist. Chiasmus is thereby also, of course, a kinesic figure: a dance step, or a figure of eight, or perhaps a running knot, which binds things together in a mobile rather than a static way, allowing for further shifts down the line (in that sense, it is unlike the formulaic closure of an epigram or conceit). Here is another instance, this time wholly unequivocal, from the final pages of Montaigne's book:

> Mais moy, d'une condition mixte, grossier ... me laisse tout lourdement aller aux plaisirs presents ... intellectuellement sensibles, sensiblement intellectuels.[16]
>
> [But as for me, being of a mixed and coarse condition ... I let myself be carried lumpishly away by the pleasures of the present moment ... [pleasures which are] intellectually palpable, palpably intellectual.]

The chiasmus requires no extended commentary here. Clearly, it is a way of imagining the mind–body relation as a unity rather than a duality, and it seems to me that this cognitive figure is essential to everything Montaigne does—everything that he thinks and writes—in the *Essais*.

Chiastic Kinesis in Maurice Scève's *Délie*

When Montaigne speaks of the kinesic force of poetry as a way of thinking, he means of course Latin poetry. The French poets, one has to infer, suffer from the slackness of the vernacular that he speaks of in "Sur des vers de Virgile." We know that he was familiar with their work, however, since he occasionally quotes Ronsard and Du Bellay. And although he never mentions Maurice Scève, he must at least have known of the *Délie*, given that it was still a major point of reference for Thomas Sébillet and others when Montaigne was a teenager. Scève's taut little *dizains*, with their Latinate vocabulary and word-order, were and are capable of delivering the very "secousse" Montaigne speaks of in the poetry sentence of I.26, and a single example will show that crossings-over of mind and body could also be imagined nearly a half-century before the chiastic formulations I have quoted above. Here is the whole *dizain*, one of the best-known and most frequently discussed examples of Scève's "metaphysical" mode of poetic thinking[17]:

> Asses plus long, qu'un Siecle Platonique
> Me fut le mois, que sans toy suis esté:
> Mais quand ton front je revis pacifique,
> Sejour treshault de toute honnesteté,
> Ou l'empire est du conseil arresté,
> Mes songes lors je creus estre devins.
> Car en mon corps: mon Ame tu revins,
> Sentant ses mains, mains celestement blanches,
> Avec leurs bras mortellement divins,
> L'un coronner mon col, l'aultre mes hanches.[18]

> [Far longer than a Platonic Year has been the month during which I have been without you: but when I saw again your pacifying brow, in which the empire of judgement is established, I believed then that my dreams were prophetic. For into my body, my Soul, you returned, feeling her hands, hands celestially white, with their arms mortally divine, one crowning my neck, the other my hips.]

Like Montaigne's formulation of the relation between mind and body, Scève's is articulated through adjectives qualified by adverbs. This grammatical patterning is, however, not in itself chiastic, as it is, for example, in the sentence "He stood there with a smile on his face, and in his hand, a rose," or indeed in the earlier quotation from Montaigne on the relation between thought and language, where the order "noun subject + complement" is inverted. In both cases, the crossing-over is effected at the semantic rather than grammatical level. However, Montaigne's "intellectuellement sensibles, sensiblement intellectuels" makes the chiasmus immediately palpable by fusing semantic inversion with lexical repetition, while Scève requires the reader, characteristically enough, to carry out inferential work in order to see that mortality is a property of the body, and thus that "mortellement" corresponds to "blanches" as "celestement" to "divins."

In Scève's *dizain*, however, the chiasmus of lines 8–9 is only one formal step within a chiastic dance performed by the last four lines, and more broadly by the poem as a whole. To speak of this movement as a dance is perhaps permissible because the embrace described in the concluding lines is similar to that of dancing partners: it has erotic implicatures, but it is also polite, elegant, stately. Line 7 already anticipates the embrace in a manner that gestures towards the chiastic: "Car en mon corps: mon Ame, tu revins." The return of soul to body enacts kinesis as a quickening, a reawakening to life, and the binding of body to soul is done by the sheer collocation of "mon corps: mon Ame." Although "mon Ame" is grammatically vocative, it affords the insertion of the noun pair "body+soul" into the centre of the line that realizes the poem's *volta*. What emerges then is something like the chiastic figure [a^1] b^1 b^2 [a^2], where [a] is grammatical wrapping rather than a semantic or lexical constant.[19]

This sounds formalistic when it is spelt out reflectively, but in the pre-reflective act of reading, it emerges as an overdetermined motor resonance: the complex act of *returning*, which is also a turning, the body towards the soul and the soul towards the body (they end up, in the embrace, face to face).[20] A key factor in the overdetermination is the implied shift in the function of the second person, which in the first six lines refers unequivocally to Délie but now, in the seventh, refers to the speaker's soul (in the eighth, "you" correspondingly becomes "she"): the whole point of the dance is that Délie is both herself (a woman with a body) and the speaker's animating spirit, his "mind." These two cross over, embrace, become a chiasmus in movement: the arm round his shoulders and the arm round his hips describe a helix, the reconciliation of the closed figure of a circle with open-ended linear motion. And since the turning of the spheres through complex circular and helical figures is resolved in a "Platonic year," the *dizain* from its opening affords a perspective in which the microcosmic chiasmus of the last four lines is embedded in a macrocosmic conceptual frame.

Scève's figurative metaphysics, as a way of thinking, is far removed from the tangible, this-wordly kinesis of Montaigne's prose. Yet the *dizain* works just as Montaigne will later say that poetry works: its *sententia*, turning on Délie's imagined "conseil" (*consilium*, *jugement*), is likewise conjoined with a sensible body in order to deliver a "secousse" that is not merely aesthetic (although it is of course that too) but fully cognitive. Like Montaigne's, Scève's is a kind of thinking that is pertinent to life as it is lived, and more particularly to the sense of life: that kinesic quickening you feel as mind turns to body and vice versa.

Kinesic Intelligence: How to Read Poetry, How to Read Montaigne

One of my objectives in juxtaposing Scève's poem with Montaigne's prose is to make a broad point about the relation of cognitive criticism to historical and cultural specificities. There is, it seems to me, no real problem here, no loss of the historical particular in some atemporal cognitive universal.[21] Human cognition is always apparent through the particular forms it adopts: the drive to inventiveness, flexibility, adaptation, just is its specialty. To which one may add the cognitive principle that any interpretation of a communicative act must, if it wants to avoid pure contingency, take account of relevant context, the changing meanings of words, possible frames of cultural reference, and so on. It follows that one could regard these two fragments as items in a virtual archive of ways of imagining the body–mind relation in the pre-Cartesian era, with the proviso, of course, that things weren't suddenly transformed by the advent of Descartes or anyone else.[22] That archive would belong to a cognitive project, not to a history of ideas or of philosophy as such: it would be made possible by the instruments of analysis that a cognitive perspective affords.

Yet our interest in reading Scève or Montaigne cannot be *purely* historical, as if their works were simply documents providing evidence of an early modern thought-world. They elicit both unreflective responses, whether kinesic, sensorimotor, affective, or indeed inferential, and reflective rereadings, higher-order analyses, evaluations, that give every appearance of being worthwhile: they reward extended consideration. That is no doubt a truism, and no one could write an essay such as this one without making some such assumption. The question, again within the cognitive perspective, lies in the particular kinds of relation between the unreflective and the reflective that these works exhibit, and more particularly in the virtually undecidable but always fascinating crossings-over between those two apparently different modes. For there is of course a critical difference at the extremes, the difference we think of as that between mind and body, body and mind; but it is essential to resist the temptation to turn the two ends of a scale or gradient into an antithesis with an excluded middle. In cognition, there is no excluded middle. The middle is the very ground on which human cognition (unlike computer cognition, for example) operates.

How, then, according to this cognitive methodology, do we read Montaigne's embodied mind, or Scève's? What kinds and degrees of kinesic intelligence may we infer from the writers' way with language, and how much of it is required to read such texts? It seems evident, to begin with, that a high degree of kinesic intelligence must be imputed to Scève, to Montaigne, and to the Latin poets Montaigne reads in "Sur des vers de Virgile." Kinesic intelligence is defined in that perspective as a highly developed feel for the kinds of language that will elicit motor responses, for the configurations of verse or prose that have "fingers." It is important to note here that kinesis gives no priority to visual representation: you may in some sense "see" the embrace described by Scève, or Montaigne's groping movement through a misty landscape, but in both instances seeing is surely only marginal, an epiphenomenon. What is essential is the motor trajectory itself, the gait, the things you can do with arms, shoulders, legs, fingers and the sensations those movements afford. Furthermore, the skills in question don't themselves belong to some privileged aesthetic category. Montaigne's prose, and even the rarefied poetic language of Scève, use *everyday* kinaesthetic processes and responses with optimal relevance, although the everyday motions of language are raised to a high level of intensity and (with Montaigne) a deceptively self-effacing control.

The notion of kinesic intelligence is helpful in such cases precisely because it doesn't pre-suppose a second-order awareness of the kind that characterizes early modern theories of the mind or soul, let alone modern cognitive science. Montaigne thought a lot about style and about language, and the special variety of prose that he wrote was in general the outcome of choices and preferences established at the earliest stages of composition of the *Essais*. But many of these were certainly what we would call "intuitive," where intuition is defined as a way of describing the pre-reflective mode: they emerged, one assumes, as a *habitus* formed by procedural memories of reading and of conversation.

The prefix "pre-" as I have been using it is designed primarily to refer to processes that do not exhibit higher-order reflection but are in some sense necessary precursors of such reflection. Such a model is complicated by the feedback loops that are a primary feature of human cognition: procedural memories based on earlier reflective episodes of the kind afforded by education are one obvious example. A whole model of how the brain marshals materials for use at a given moment of engagement with the world is involved here, and this is not the place to explore it further, but it is essential to bear in mind that the economy of cognition is fundamentally temporal, and that reminder is usefully provided by the prefix "pre-."[23]

In short, then, I would propose a definition of kinesic intelligence that avoids assigning any kind of necessarily reflective awareness to "intelligence." The phrase would of course not be appropriate to describe a programmed motor response of the kind exhibited in the behaviour of flocks of birds, shoals of fish, and some football crowds (the Mexican wave, for example): "kinesis" on its own is adequate there. But as soon as the motor response enters into a network of other kinds of response, especially (in our context) linguistic ones, variable skills of discrimination and interpretation begin to manifest themselves, whether pre-reflectively or reflectively. Kinesic intelligence is, from the bottom up, a way of thinking with the body.

It goes without saying that these remarks are equally valid for the attribution of kinesic intelligence to the reader. Motor resonance is typically, after all, a shared experience, although not, in most cases, a reciprocal one (which is one of the reasons why the expression "mirror neurons" can be misleading). Montaigne's kinesic intelligence provides him with a powerful instrument for creating effects in the reader, but if we, as readers, are to experience those effects, we need not only the primary resources of motor resonance but also the linguistic knowledge, skills and experience that mediate the resonance.

That means, in turn, that allowance needs to be made for considerable readerly variation. Over the centuries, many people have read the opening pages of "De l'institution des enfans": it was from the outset one of the most popular chapters of the *Essais*. Were they all conscious of the effects we have been addressing here? Certainly not. Have they all felt them unconsciously (unreflectively or pre-reflectively)? Arguably they must have at some level, even if the spectrum of cognitive preferences and responses to language varies very widely. I want to propose that, for any close reader, they would have been significantly operative at the pre-reflective level:

they would have affected the way the meaning was grasped. No doubt for many other readers they have been purely residual, and if someone pointed them out, they would say that the kinesis was only a trivial side-effect. I would be inclined to say that in that case the cognitive preferences (or cultural habits) of the reader would have acted to close down the responses, regard them as irrelevant, but that it would be impossible to read the passage at all if they were absent. How could they be absent? The language can't do its work without them.

The handful of texts we have been considering here are explicitly about cognition across its whole range, from the inflections of intelligent thought and language, via imagination, to the habitual gait of the body or the sensorimotor reach required in order to perform an embrace, and back again. That is in itself hardly surprising: both Montaigne and Scève are known to be writers who actively and explicitly engage the cognitive imagination of the reader in their very different ways. The *Délie* and the *Essais* are in their entirety about cognition, its modalities, its constraints, its deficiencies, its opportunities, its habits. And they are both mobile works, crossing over ceaselessly between the mind and the body, the reflective and the sensorimotor modes, the *intellectuel* and the *sensible*. The mind, in both cases, is embodied, but through language, the body becomes a palpable mind (clearly nobody is going to say that Montaigne or Scève is just an unthinking body). The feedback loop between the reflective, the pre-reflective, and the unreflective in these texts has precisely the structure of a chiasmus.

Notes

1. See Guillemette Bolens, *Le Style des gestes: Corporéité et kinésie dans le récit littéraire* (Lausanne: Éditions BHMS, 2008; English version: *The Style of Gestures: Embodiment and Cognition in Literary Narrative*, Baltimore: Johns Hopkins University Press, 2012). Bolens acknowledges the importance of Ellen Spolsky's founding article, "Elaborated knowledge: reading kinesis in pictures," *Poetics Today* 17 (1996): 157–80.
2. I offer a less explicitly cognitive reading of this same passage, and of passages from *Essais* III.5 ("Sur des vers de Virgile"), in my essay "The Transit of Venus: Feeling Your Way Forward," in *Montaigne in Transit: Essays in Honour of Ian Maclean*, ed. Neil Kenny, Richard Scholar and Wes Williams (Oxford: Legenda, 2016), 9–18. The two readings are designed to complement one another.
3. Michel de Montaigne, *Les Essais*, ed. Pierre Villey and V.-Louis Saulnier (Paris: PUF, 1965), 146 (I.26); this reference is valid for the whole of the

passage discussed here. For the purposes of this discussion, I cite the 1580 text without the later additions in order to recover the initial dynamic of the text, and also to avoid complications and deviations into issues that are not essential here. All translations in this essay are my own.

4. It is customary to gloss Montaigne's mention of nail-biting with a reference to Horace's *Satires* I, x; but the point here must be that, even if Montaigne reflectively remembered that literary instance and meant to echo it, it is only meaningful to him and to the reader if the sensorimotor echo is triggered. In other words, the sensorimotor trumps what used to be referred to as the "intertextual."
5. For a detailed account of "tonus" and its role in literary works, see Guillemette Bolens, *L'Humour et le savoir des corps: Don Quichotte, Tristram Shandy et le rire du lecteur* (Rennes: Presses Universitaires de Rennes, 2016). The term (more common in French than in English) refers to muscle tone, or, more specifically, a normal state of continuous slight tension in muscle tissue that facilitates its response to stimulation.
6. Spolsky, "Elaborated Knowledge," 159.
7. "Implicature" is an implication that the speaker intends the interlocutor to derive. This term, like "procedural expression" used below, is adapted broadly speaking from relevance theory, a theory of communication that insists on the dynamic character of communicative utterances, and on the extent to which they elicit from the interlocutor a reciprocal activity. See my study *Thinking with Literature: Towards a Cognitive Criticism* (Oxford: Oxford University Press, 2016), especially 24–6 and chs 3 and 6.
8. For a technical account of the conceptual/procedural distinction (proposed by Diane Blakemore), see Robyn Carston, *Thoughts and Utterances: The Pragmatics of Explicit Communication* (Oxford: Blackwell, 2002), 160–4.
9. "Thinking on the wing" is an expression designed to capture the dynamic character of language in use, in other words the way in which relevance theory thinks about language.
10. On rethinking the "metaphorical" and the "literal" in response to embodied cognition, see Kathryn Banks in this volume.
11. "Et, entreprenant de parler …" (146).
12. "The Transit of Venus," 11–13.
13. I have wanted to avoid "self-expression" as a rendering of "s'expliquer" for reasons that will perhaps be obvious: Montaigne is not talking about the personal, confessional mode here; "s'expliquer" has the sense of "getting across one's meaning," "making oneself clear." Communication of thoughts is what is at issue here, not the expression of feelings, etc.
14. I have added quotation marks simply in order to make the structure of the chiasmus immediately apparent.

15. The imagination is already, in the sixteenth century, associated with a quasi-Platonic ascent whereby the corporality of material things is "raised up" towards conceptual understanding. In later ages, this upwards movement will become associated with balloon flight: see *Thinking with Literature*, chs 3 and 5.
16. *Essais*, III.13 ("De l'experience"), 1107.
17. The ascription of Scève's poetry to the category of the metaphysical (in the sense used for the poetry of John Donne and others) was first made, as far as I am aware, by Odette de Mourgues in her study *Metaphysical, Baroque and Précieux Poetry* (Oxford: The Clarendon Press, 1953), 110–25; for her analysis of the *dizain* I discuss here, see 21–2. The *dizain* has been revisited many times since; this is not the place to provide a bibliographical review.
18. *The "Délie" of Maurice Scève*, ed. I.D. McFarlane (Cambridge: Cambridge University Press, 1966), 320 (*dizain* 367).
19. On the possibilities offered by the *dizain* form, see my article "Rime et structure du dizain dans la *Délie* de Maurice Scève," in *Les Fruits de la saison. Mélanges de Littérature des XVIe et XVIIe siècles offerts au Professeur André Gendre*, ed. Philippe Terrier, Loris Petris, Marie-Jeanne Liengme Bessire (Geneva: Droz, 2000), 49–57 (56–7 for a discussion of the chiastic figures in *dizain* 367).
20. See Ullrich Langer's essay in this volume on Virgil's lovers turning towards each other, and on more or less embodied versions of this scenario in later poets including Scève.
21. This objection continues to be made, despite rebuttals and counter-examples in a number of recent publications; these include Alan Richardson, *The Neural Sublime: Cognitive Theories and Romantic Texts* (Baltimore: Johns Hopkins, 2010), Introduction; Mark J. Bruhn and Donald R. Wehrs, eds, *Cognition, Literature, and History* (New York: Routledge, 2014); and my essay "Situated cognition: the literary archive," in *Poetics Today* 38 (2017): 235–53. See also the Introduction to this volume, pp.1–12
22. Andrew Marvell's poem "The Garden," probably composed in the 1660s in a different country and a different language, is another item for the archive: see my brief discussion of two stanzas from the poem in *"Far Other Worlds and Other Seas": Thinking with Literature in the Twenty-First Century*, the sixth annual lecture of the International Balzan Foundation (Milan: Olschki, 2015), also in "Situated cognition" (see above, n. 21), pp. 248–50). Cf also John Donne's "The Ecstasy."
23. The point is valid also within the macro-perspective of evolution, where a gradual emergence of human reflective capacity from mental processes anticipating or affording that capacity (providing a platform for it) needs to be assumed. Early hominin cognition in general, one might say, was characterized by pre-reflective processes. For a more extended discussion of the relation between pre-reflective and reflective cognition, see *Thinking with Literature*, especially 21–4, 40–2.

Bibliography

Bolens, Guillemette. *Le Style des gestes: Corporéité et kinésie dans le récit littéraire*. Lausanne: Éditions BHMS, 2008. Translated as: *The Style of Gestures: Embodiment and Cognition in Literary Narrative*. Baltimore: Johns Hopkins University Press, 2012.

———. *L'Humour et le savoir des corps: Don Quichotte, Tristram Shandy et le rire du lecteur*. Rennes: Presses Universitaires de Rennes, 2016.

Bruhn, Mark J., and Donald R. Wehrs, eds, *Cognition, Literature, and History*. New York: Routledge, 2014.

Carston, Robyn. *Thoughts and Utterances: The Pragmatics of Explicit Communication*. Oxford: Blackwell, 2002.

Cave, Terence. Rime et structure du dizain dans la *Délie* de Maurice Scève. In *Les Fruits de la saison. Mélanges de Littérature des XVIe et XVIIe siècles offerts au Professeur André Gendre*, edited by Philippe Terrier, Loris Petris, Marie-Jeanne Liengme Bessire, 49–57. Geneva: Droz, 2000.

———. *"Far Other Worlds and Other Seas": Thinking with Literature in the Twenty-First Century*. The Sixth Annual Lecture of the International Balzan Foundation. Milan: Olschki, 2015.

———. *Thinking with Literature: Towards a Cognitive Criticism*. Oxford: Oxford University Press, 2016a.

———. The Transit of Venus: Feeling Your Way Forward. In *Montaigne in Transit: Essays in Honour of Ian Maclean*, edited by Neil Kenny, Richard Scholar and Wes Williams, 9–18. Oxford: Legenda, 2016b.

———. Situated Cognition: The Literary Archive. In *Poetics Today* 38 (2017): 235–53.

de Montaigne, Michel. *Les Essais*. Edited by Pierre Villey and Verdun-Louis Saulnier. Paris: PUF, 1965.

de Mourgues, Odette. *Metaphysical, Baroque and Précieux Poetry*. Oxford: The Clarendon Press, 1953.

Richardson, Alan. *The Neural Sublime: Cognitive Theories and Romantic Texts*. Baltimore: Johns Hopkins University Press, 2010.

Scève, Maurice. *The "Délie."* Edited by I. D. McFarlane. Cambridge: Cambridge University Press, 1966.

Spolsky, Ellen. Elaborated Knowledge: Reading Kinesis in Pictures. *Poetics Today* 17 (1996): 157–80.

CHAPTER 3

Turning Toward the Beloved (Virgil, Petrarch, Scève)

Ullrich Langer

Three poems—a section of Virgil's fourth *Georgic*, a sonnet by Petrarch, and a *dizain* by Maurice Scève—will constitute my brief demonstration of kinesic intelligence at the heart of one of the most enduring scenarios in early modern lyric poetry. Although they are in a chronological sequence, and the later authors knew the earlier poems, neither Petrarch's sonnet nor Scève's *dizain* are a discernible *reading* of the earlier poem or poems. It is more my contention that the physical scenario in Virgil is a powerful archetypal incarnation of the gestures underlying and conveying the designation of the beloved, and I understand the later poems to be versions of this designation. Read on the background of the Virgil fragment, Petrarch's and Scève's poems are also demonstrations of how these gestures become absorbed into other, less directly physical, levels of literary representation. Even in the Virgilian scenario itself, it is impossible to segregate physical movement from the various meanings derived from its representation, and that integration of the physical into the semantically complex makes it no less powerful.

Indeed, the representation of physical gesture in these samples—the turning of Orpheus to Eurydice, and her stretching out toward him—is

U. Langer (✉)
University of Wisconsin-Madison, Madison, WI, USA

K. Banks, T. Chesters (eds.), *Movement in Renaissance Literature*, Cognitive Studies in Literature and Performance, https://doi.org/10.1007/978-3-319-69200-5_3

hardly distinguishable from other layers in the "discourse" of (lyric) poetry, and particularly figures of rhetoric, such as the apostrophe, and the shift from a universal cause to an individual cause. Gesture seems to be the physical origin, as it were, of these discursive phenomena, as if gesture echoed in various ways throughout the representation. The intentionality of the initial gesture is reinforced by the successive literary correlations to the physical gesture, both in the Virgilian passage itself and in the later poems. Although each of these is further removed from the physical movement as such and from its direct perception in the diegesis by the beloved (Eurydice or Orpheus), the intentions that the movement manifested are absorbed into, and made explicit, by various features of the later literary representations.

My more specific claims are the following: the turning toward an object of love is a gesture of designation or intention, in accordance with love's idealization of the beloved.[1] The movement toward the beloved is also a sign of life[2]; it confirms (and, ironically, ruins) the presumed victory over death. The turn toward the beloved provokes an empathic movement on the part of the reader/listener. This empathic movement is central to an implicit conceptual argument made, at least in the Virgil segment: it undergirds the plea for equity, in the form of pardon, on the background of a harsh law. However, the language used to represent the response of the beloved complicates—both strengthening and weakening—the implicit legal case. In the poems by Petrarch and Scève, the gesture of turning-toward resonates as a shift from universal to particular address. A similar implicit case for equity (in the form of pardon) can be made, with similarly predictable tragic results.

> Iamque pedem referens casus evaserat omnis,
> redditaque Eurydice superas veniebat ad auras,
> pone sequens (namque hanc dederat Proserpina legem),
> cum subita incautum dementia cepit amantem,
> ignoscenda quidem, scirent si ignoscere Manes:
> restitit, Eurydicenque suam iam luce sub ipsa
> immemor heu ! victusque animi respexit. ibi omnis
> effusus labor atque immitis rupta tyranni
> foedera, terque fragor stagnis auditus Avernis.
> illa 'quis et me' inquit 'miseram et te perdidit, Orpheu,
> quis tantus furor ? en iterum crudelia retro
> fata vocant conditque natantia lumina somnus.
> iamque vale: feror ingenti circumdata nocte

invalidasque tibi tendens, heu ! non tua, palmas.'[3]
(*Georgics*, IV, 485–499)

[And now, as he retraced his steps, he had avoided all accident, and the returned Eurydice was nearing the upper air, following behind (for Proserpina had given that law), when a sudden madness seized the imprudent lover, to be pardoned, indeed, if the shades knew how to pardon: he halted, and on the very verge of light, forgetful, alas, and his mind vanquished, he looked back at his Eurydice. In that instant all the labour was spilled and the pacts of the savage tyrant were broken, and three times a peal of thunder was heard among the pools of Avernus. She cried, "who has ruined me, woeful, and you, Orpheus, what immense frenzy? look, again the cruel fates call [me] back, and sleep seals my swimming eyes. And now farewell: I am borne away, surrounded by a vast night, and stretching my strengthless palms to you—alas, not yours."][4]

The final, tragic encounter of Orpheus and Eurydice consists of movements, at the core of which are two specific gestures.[5] Orpheus stops and turns around to look at Eurydice. Eurydice stretches her arms toward her husband before she is pulled back into Hades. Especially at the outset Virgil fills these lines with indications of movement—*pedem referens*, *evaserat*, *veniebat*, *sequens*, *restitit*, *respixit*—referring to the lovers. But other expressions are also (originally) indications of movement, and function as a catachresis: most notably *reddita Eurydice*, Eurydice *given* back, as Proserpina had *given* the law, *dederat legem*.[6] Frenzy overtaking Orpheus is worded as "frenzy *seized* him," *dementia cepit*. The scenario and the negotiations that allowed this to happen are all suffused with taking and giving humans and things. All aspects of this scene are meant to provoke the response of empathy that kinesic intelligence insists upon. We know Orpheus and Eurydice because their gestures toward each other are the result of other such gestures, taking them away and giving them back. Our empathic imitation of their final failed tending toward each other is all the deeper since it can rely on layers of such movement, a kind of kinesic memory.[7]

* * *

Virgil waters down the final indications of movement: *effusus*, *natantia*, *feror*, *circumdata*. Spilled, swimming, born away, surrounded. In the midst of these, surrounded by these weaker evocations of movement (although *circumdata* is an ironic reminder of the earlier *reddita* and *dederat*) is the strong *tendens palmas*: the stretching of the hands that point to and cannot reach the lover. This last gesture of Eurydice is indeed singular, not to be repeated. The passivity and diffuseness of the later movements correspond to her slow drifting-back into Hades, and her transformation into a shade.

The gestures of tending to the other articulate kinetically the belongingness of the two persons to each other, and function for the lovers as kinesic markers of their love. When Orpheus looks back, he does so to look at *Eurydicen suam*, and when Eurydice addresses her husband, she reiterates this possession, as something no longer possible: *heu! non tua*. The agent of *tendens palmas* is quite literally *non tua*. In addition, she invokes the couple's intimacy, through their shared perdition, in the parallelism *et me … et te*. Intimacy but also acknowledgement of their separation, and of the different forms that their ruin will take: she does not ask *quis nos perdidit* but *quis et me … et te perdidit*? The language she chooses mimics the pulling apart that is already taking place physically.[8]

The gesture of tending toward the beloved impels a mimetic response from the reader, in the obvious sense of an understanding of the desire for the beloved, the *only* beloved. We understand what it means to turn toward a specific person, and behind that gesture and that desire, we sense all of the steps that Orpheus needed to perform in order to arrive at this point. The turning toward does not convey a general love for women or men, but the sense that this particular individual is being designated, this particular love is being singled out. Our empathic understanding trains us, as it were, to perform this designation of the particular case. In other words, the gesture of Orpheus prepares us to pardon him, as it performs what we need to perform (and what the shades do not know how to perform, because they are not human). Orpheus and Eurydice should be an exception.

Virgil's passage furnishes us with elements of a legal case for pardon, as an act of equity. First, through the suspended identification by Eurydice of who is responsible for his turning:

> illa 'quis et me' inquit 'miseram et te perdidit, Orpheu,
> quis tantus furor ? …

Quis, in its first instance, is apparently an interrogative pronoun ("who?"), and only in the next line is understood as an interrogative adjective modifying *furor* ("what frenzy?"). It is as if Orpheus were exculpated, separated from his amorous frenzy, by its victim. Who did this to me and to you? (It was someone other than you). Furthermore, the scene is replete with juridical language. Proserpina has laid down a "law" (*dederat … legem*)[9]; the law concerns possession of Eurydice: she was "returned," *reddita*, to her husband, becoming *his*, but when Orpheus breaks the agreement, she becomes no longer *his*, and she is summoned by the fates (*fata vocant*). Orpheus's *dementia* is to be pardoned, *ignoscenda*, if only the shades knew how to pardon, *ignoscere*. The lover's looking back breaks the pacts, *rupta … foedera*, of the savage tyrant. When Eurydice invokes her husband's *furor*, she describes someone who, according to Roman law and the (later) *Institutes*, would not have been in a position to be partner to a contract.[10] If the shades "knew" how to pardon, they would have pardoned Orpheus. In addition, we the readers would have pardoned Orpheus, in this specific instance, as our kinaesthetic understanding of Orpheus's gesture has trained us to do.[11] The re-enactment of the gesture of specific intention is a cognitive activity, not the link to a fixed idea already in place. We have gained knowledge of lovers' frenzy through this specific re-enactment, not because someone has told us that all lovers are mad, but because we have turned, as well, to Eurydice. As a Renaissance commentator, Filippo Venuti, repeats,

> [S]e conoscessimo quanto ardentemente, & miserabilmente desiderano gli innamorati di vedere la cosa amata, & quanto sia vehemente questa perturbatione in tal cosa, giudicariamo quelli meritare ogni perdono in tale errore: ma l'ombre infernali per la loro crudeltà, non hanno mai conosciuta alcuna humanità.[12]
>
> [If we knew how ardently and miserably lovers desire to see the beloved, and how violent their trouble is in such things, we would judge that they merit pardon for such an error, but the infernal shades, because of their cruelty, have never known any such sense of humanity.]

We *do* know, now, how lovers act. Indeed, the "aspra, & iniqua legge" ["harsh and inequitable law"] (ibid.)[13] of the savage tyrant, of the shades and of the cruel fates, should have allowed for an exception, here in this instance. This exception to the severe law is motivated by *humanità*, by a sense of gentleness that is achieved by knowing what lovers experience, by putting yourself in their place. In legal terms, the exception made for Orpheus and Eurydice would have been called "equity" (*aequitas*, *epieikeia*), an attention to the particular case that should not be judged under an overly severe or rigid law. The gestures of the tragic lovers demonstrate, render palpable, the "frenzy" that overtook Orpheus. In addition, his turning around manifested visibly his violation of the law given by Proserpina, since he did not continue on the path as directed by the "tyrant." This gesture—and the stretching of the wife's hands toward her husband—allow us to assimilate the knowledge of the *subita dementia* that vanquished Orpheus's prudence, and that should have occasioned a judgment of equity, an exception to the *aspra legge*.[14] These gestures also incarnate the turn toward the particular as an ethical value, as an attentiveness to the singular case that calls for an exception to the law.

Following Orpheus's turn and accompanying or preceding her own stretching out to him is Eurydice's address. It is an *apostrophe*, a specific address, and not a general complaint about her or their misfortune; it is the vocative *Orpheu* that ends the line.[15] The turning of her speech toward her husband corresponds to his turning around to look at her. She does not address the cruel fates, or Proserpina, but her impassioned lover, at the moment of falling back into the pools of Avernus. This is an address of extreme specificity: it is only you I address, no one else. This might seem trite to us, but it reinforces all the gestural mise-en-scène: the turning around to look at one person, the tending of the palms to one person. It also reinforces the juridical case for pardon. This is a specific, exceptional case in which the harsh law should not be applied.

But one can argue that the exceptional couple's case is not specific: as Venuti observed, following the commentary tradition, all (true) lovers are dominated by a *dementia*, a *furor*.[16] Our sense that Orpheus and Eurydice should be pardoned relies on our universal knowledge about the behaviour of lovers. However the frenzy, the *pazzia*, of lovers is precisely the (no doubt mistaken) feeling that no one else will ever do, that the beloved cannot be substituted for, that there would be absolutely no consolation if she were lost. The scenario of Orpheus and Eurydice stages a feeling about another person as entirely unique; the lovers themselves would not, at the moments of greatest intensity of longing, universalize their feeling: it is only me and you, *et me … et te*.[17] And yet this scenario of uniqueness, of utter specificity, is staged as accessible to all (humane) readers, looking on from the outside. It is the gestures that initiate us into the resistance of that specificity to harsh laws, and provide a kind of pre-rational unlocking of our sense of the necessity for pardon.

Before moving to my next sample, I need to acknowledge how this coherent scenario (turning-toward—empathy—equity—pardon) is rendered more complex by Virgil, and the love of the famous couple is less unified than I suggested. Eurydice is the only one who speaks, and in her speech, her apostrophe, while allowing for exculpation or at least pardon, as we have seen, she nevertheless points out the disastrous consequences of his mindless gesture. Virgil characterizes her final gesture as *tendens palmas*.[18] The palms are a synecdoche for the hands, which is not unusual, but Virgil's word is ambiguous, since *palmae* are also the branches or leaves of a palm tree, and a common symbol of victory, as the expressions *palmam deferre* or *palmam ferre* attest.[19] Eurydice is handing Orpheus his impotent or useless victories: his poetic conquest of Hades has been undone by his transgression of Proserpina's law. Palms are then an ironic choice; Orpheus has earned defeat, not victory. I, Eurydice, should be the symbol of your victory over death and am offering you the palms of your victory that you cannot hold yourself. The "palms" are tragic and pathetic, marking the abyss between what he could have achieved and what he did not achieve, by his own doing. In this sense the rhetorical fashioning of the scenario undermines the case for pardon, and blocks or makes more difficult our empathic understanding of Orpheus's gesture.

This blockage occurs not at the level of kinesic knowledge, not as a conflicting physical re-enactment, but at a discursive level (the understanding of the symbol of victory that are the palms): the literary scenario, in this case, prevents us from easily moving from kinesic intelligence to all other levels of the representation. Tending "palms" toward another is, on the level of kinesic intelligence, an attempt to join the other (in love), to reduce the physical distance between the bodies. When, however, the ironic sense of the word "palms" becomes clear to us, the separation between the two bodies is emphasized, not reduced. In addition, the choice of "palms" introduces the presence of the poet, the consciousness of someone emphasizing the futility of Eurydice's gesture, while the kinetic elements of the scene all support the joining of the lovers. This might very well be a feature of irony in general, and certainly of Virgil's irony in particular.

* * *

Another such scenario can be found in Petrarch's *Rime sparse*. It is deprived of the explicit kinetic elements, the turning-around and the stretching-toward, that made the Orpheus-Eurydice scene so intensely pathetic. Instead, I will argue that the kinetic elements are transposed into a move from the universal to the particular, and manifested in the apostrophe.

In addition, the gesture of turning subtends, as it were, the sonnet, as a memory of the *rivolta d'occhi* (the turning of the eyes, the glance) that earlier occasioned the lover's ecstasy. The lover can no longer turn his eyes to her but he can turn his speech to her. The sonnet in question is the first to come after the poet has learned of the death of his beloved, and it begins what many editions have marked as the second part of the *Canzoniere*. *Rime sparse* 267 is punctuated by a series of exclamations, followed by an apostrophe, an injunction to the poet himself, and a memory of a strangely evanescent encounter with Laura:

> Oimè il bel viso, oimè il soave sguardo,
> oimè il leggiadro portamento altero;
> oimè il parlar ch'ogni aspro ingegno et fero
> facevi humile, ed ogni huom vil gagliardo!
> et oimè il dolce riso, onde uscìo 'l dardo
> di che morte, altro bene omai non spero:
> alma real, dignissima d'impero,
> se non fossi fra noi scesa sì tardo!
> Per voi conven ch'io arda, e 'n voi respire,
> ch'i' pur fui vostro; et se di voi son privo,
> via men d'ogni sventura altra mi dole.
> Di speranza m'empieste et di desire,
> quand'io partì' dal sommo piacer vivo;
> ma 'l vento ne portava le parole.[20]

> [Alas the lovely face, alas the gentle glance, alas the proud, carefree bearing! Alas the speech that made every harsh or savage mind humble and every base man valiant!
> And alas the sweet smile whence came forth the dart from which now I expect death, no other good! Regal soul, worthy of all empire if you had not come down among us so late:
> for you I must burn, in you breathe, for I have been only yours; and if I am deprived of you, it pains me more than any other misfortune;
> with hope you filled me and with desire, when I left still alive that highest pleasure, but the wind carried off the words.]

Petrarch's praise of Laura, and his lament of her loss, are formulated in terms of a *descent* of the beloved among us.[21] As Orpheus descended into Hades to retrieve Eurydice, so does Laura descend from the heavens, it is implied, into the sublunary sphere among all of us on earth. Similarly to Orpheus, again, Laura's *katábasis* is a failure; it has happened too late, despite her victories over proud men, over the "harsh" ("aspro") and the savage ("fero"). Orpheus, too, vanquished the savage with his sweet voice and he was able to triumph over the harshest of all laws, death, with the power of that voice.

If the tragic last encounter between Orpheus and Eurydice is represented through the reciprocal gestures of the couple, no such gestures are featured as Petrarch the lover laments the taking away of Laura. The sonnet consists of speech praising Laura and a specific address to Laura's soul. The praise of the attributes of Laura (l. 1–6) is introduced by the exclamation "oimè," manifesting here the sighs from which he "nourished his heart" (*Rime sparse* 1, l. 2), and an expression of pure emotion, of extreme pre-linguistic intimacy.[22] The expression of that emotion as part of the praise of Laura allows the reader to share it, and its common occurrence as a sign of lamentation points to its universal nature. The very fact that the anaphoric quasi-onomatopoeia is imitated from the poetry of a near-contemporary, Cino da Pistoia, speaks to the universal nature of loss and grief. Similarly, the lexical elements of the first six lines (*viso*, *sguardo*, *portamento*, *parlar*, *riso*) are no surprise to readers of love lyric—and why should they be? Much of the preceding poetry in the *Canzoniere* has praised these features of Laura's appearance, and it would be strange if their loss did not elicit anything but anguish. That anguish seems all the greater in that *all* men were made better—humbled if they were arrogant, lifted up if they were base—by her speech that formed a harmony with her face, glance, bearing, and smile.

This is what poetry, under the classic rhetorical model, is supposed to do: demonstrate how the existence of Laura, that particular, limited case, had an effect on all men, and acceded to a value that is shared by all. It is the passage of a *causa finita* to a *causa infinita*, in rhetorical terms,[23] and proper to poetry; this is confirmed by Aristotle in his *Poetics* (1451a36–1451b11), but more relevantly to Petrarch, by Cicero in the *Pro Archia*; as poetry is embedded in what links the humane disciplines to each other, it has the function of addressing universal themes, and it provides solace and refuge in times of adversity.[24] The definite article introducing the different features of Laura, "*il* bel viso … *il* soave sguardo … *il* leggiadro portamento altero," and so forth, contrasts with what we can sometimes find in other contexts, *these* beautiful eyes (for example, "*questi* son *que'* begli occhi," 75, l. 9 and 12). It is not only as if the poet were making them available to all, but by lifting them out of the instant and the circumstance that are indicated elsewhere in the collection by the demonstrative, he is also lending them a duration they do not have when they are tied to an encounter in a specific moment. The definite article also, obviously, contrasts with the possessive: it is *the* lovely face and not *your* lovely face. Death and poetry allows your beauty to no longer be yours, but everyone's. This is all the more poignant in that the second half of the sonnet personalizes the lament to an extreme, in an attempt to reappropriate Laura to herself and to her lover: *voi* and *vostro* and *io* are strewn about the lines (although the second-person plural's reference is not unambiguous). Finally, the definite article throughout the first five lines is masculine singular, not the feminine, expressing a kind of monumental neutral that enshrines the sweet features of Laura.

Then Petrarch turns away from a general praise of attributes as he addresses the "regal" soul of Laura and concludes his second exclamation. It is an apostrophe, in the true rhetorical sense of the word, a turning-away from all others to one in particular.[25] The soul does not really summarize all previous features of Laura, although the "civilizing" effect of her beauty and her proud bearing suggest a value that transcends the erotic. The fact that her soul is being "turned-to" is a sign of the fact that she is dead, that her body is no longer connected to her soul.[26] The soul is and was most worthy of *impero*, supreme power and the empire over which it is exercised. It is here that the lingering, and later in the collection, much more explicit, resonances of praise of the Virgin Mary, are the strongest.[27]

After a lament and praise that insist on the link between Laura and all men, the tercets return to the personal affective register, and specifically to the longing and desire that were at the heart of the poet's relationship to her. Petrarch fills the tercets with indications of the first person singular, but he chooses to address not the soul alone (since in that case he would have continued to use the second-person singular, as in *fossi*), but instead addresses the attributes he listed in the quatrains, in addition to the soul: "Per *voi* conven ch'io arda …" (l. 9).[28] The lover expands his address to include all attributes of Laura, not simply her soul, no doubt because these visual attributes and this soul together constituted the last *sommo piacer vivo*, the final and highest pleasure of their (final) encounter, which filled him with hope and desire. The wind took forth the words that produced or expressed this pleasure, most likely words spoken by Laura.

In his excellent commentary on the *Rime sparse*, Lodovico Castelvetro notes the shift from the initial enumeration and lament to the more personal tone in the tercets. He prefaces this sonnet with what could be called an *argumentum*:

> Lamento della perdita, che ha fatta per la morte di L. Annovera prima partitamente i beni perduti nella morte di L. il viso, lo sguardo, il portamento, il parlare, il riso. Poi, perche la perdita di questi beni pareva commune a tutti, rivolge il parlare all'anima di L. & le dice, che a lui tocca piu di piangere, che a gli altri, che fu amato da lei. & se n'avide nelle promesse fattegli, quando si parti da lei. le quali per questa morte sono tornate vane.[29]
>
> [A lament of the loss that he has experienced with the death of Laura. He will list first bit by bit the lost goods in the death of Laura, the face, the glance, the bearing, the speech, the smile. Then, because the loss of these goods seemed common to all, he turns his speech to the soul of Laura and tells her, that it is more up to him to weep, than to the others, since he was loved by her, and he realizes this in the promises that were made to him, when he left her, which because of this death were made vain.]

Since the "goods" that constituted Laura's appearance and bearing and speech were appreciable by all, and their loss shared by all ("commune a tutti"), the lament of their loss is not somehow sufficient. The loss of a great leader or the loss of an abundant country can be lamented effectively by anyone, since the leader's actions benefited many and the abundant country nourished many; the leader was great in that his actions produced goods for many, not in that he had a particularly loving relationship with his family, and so forth. So one laments in the great leader the effect of his actions for the many, not, except incidentally, his love for his family. But in this case the relationship between Petrarch and Laura is that which makes the lament appropriate. It is that which needs to be added. The fact that the lover's specific loss completes, perfects, the lament means that in the end, it is that loss that *really* counts, and it is that loss that is truly felt, that can be expressed in concrete terms. The shift of the lament from the "common goods" to the soul—why, by the way, should the soul not be counted among the goods appreciated by all?—and the refocusing of the lament to a past personal exchange of words and glances is a movement from the general to the particular, a move that excludes all others from this intense loss, and that also, by this very exclusion, makes the lament the most powerful of all. Castelvetro uses the verb *rivolgere* ("rivolge il parlare")[30]: the poet turns his speech, in the gesture that is the apostrophe, to her soul as a lover turns to his only beloved. The commentator has used the same word as Petrarch himself used to designate Laura's glance, *una rivolta d'occhi* (72, ll. 34–35), a glance that precipitates the ecstatic experience of joy ("Vaghe faville, angeliche, beatrici…," l. 37) in one of the most famous of the *Rime sparse*'s *canzoni*. Petrarch turns, "rivolge," his speech to Laura in her death as she had turned to look at him in life. It is this turn, and the glance, that are important, the specific and exclusive turning-toward that a human being and a poem can enact, not a list of qualities that constitute the "goods" lost in her death.

The existential intention that distinguishes Petrarch's lament from the common rhetoric of praise is also a feature of the initial encounter between poet and (future) beloved. The lament is a glance to Laura as her glancing at him set off the radical change in his life that was his love. Lamentation recuperates the initial turning-toward that is the beginning of passion and the existential source of the *Canzoniere*; this over-determination, or over-laying of mourning and passion, is made possible by the shift from the commonly shared to the utterly particular.

As in the retrieval of Eurydice from the underworld, the particular case is set against a cruel law, although in Petrarch's lament this is not made explicit. The cruel law is, of course, the universal grip of death, that law that suffers no exception.[31] Petrarch's turning toward Laura is a movement in speech that allows us to sense the need for pardon, for attentiveness to the particular faced with the harsh universal, and pardon is just as unlikely to be given.

* * *

My final example is further yet removed from the Orpheus-Eurydice scenario, and a step beyond Petrarch, in that it is not a lament of a deceased beloved, but both a praise of a living beloved and a lament occasioned by the suffering that the love for her produces in the poet-lover. In this case, it is an implied *katábasis*, a descent of the beloved, perfected by God, into this world, and it moves from the hyperbolic universal to the extreme particular. Maurice Scève's *Delie, object de plus haulte vertu* (1544) is the first of many Petrarch-inspired collections in the French lyric tradition that elide the beloved's death. The relevant *dizain* is inspired by many sources, Neoplatonic as well as Petrarchan:

> Le Naturant par ses haultes Idées
> Rendit de soy la Nature admirable.
> Par les vertus de sa vertu guidées
> S'esvertua en œuvre esmerveillable.
> Car de tout bien, voyre es Dieux desirable,
> Parfeit un corps en sa perfection,

> Mouvant aux Cieulx telle admiration,
> Qu'au premier œil mon ame l'adora,
> Comme de tous la delectation
> Et de moy seul fatale Pandora.[32]

> [The maker of Nature [God] by his elevated Ideas/Rendered Nature admirable by itself (or through him)./Guided by the virtues of his virtue/He (or Nature) endeavoured in a wondrous work./For out of all goods, desirable even to the gods,/He (or Nature) perfected a body in its perfection,/ Producing in the heavens such admiration,/That at the first glance my soul adored it,/As for all an object of delectation,/And for me alone a fatal Pandora.]

A creature, fully finished, perfected by God, and furnished with all the "goods" that are admired by all, even the gods, descends, it is implied, into humanity and its sight is the delectation of all but one. The poem evokes the heights of heaven (and the Ideas)—*ses haultes Idées*—and ends with Pandora, the gifts given to humanity here on earth. The poet-lover first adores Délie with his soul, after one glance only, and then adds that in distinction to all others, for him this adoration is both a destiny and something fatal, a gift of evils. Virgil's turning, Petrarch's turning of the eyes and of speech, have become distilled, as it were, into the conceptual movement from *tous* (all) to *moy seul* (me alone). The poem's beginning expresses the beloved's praiseworthiness—that which all can admire—as a *figura etymologica*, playing on different versions of "virtue": *vertus-vertu-esvertua*. This web of universally lauded attributes extends to further polyptotons, *parfait-perfection*, *admirable-admiration*, as if the entire fabric of nature and of nature's creator were coherent evidence of her goodness. The poet is the only exception: goods to all others, evils to him. Love in this sense is precisely *not* a virtue, it is *not* something worthy of praise. This is the turning-toward that signifies the frenzy of love, the *furor* that Eurydice identifies in Orpheus and that has caused her to be lost to her husband and to fall back to Hades. The same frenzy enabled Orpheus to vanquish death, and it is the same frenzy that exculpates him, that is a cause for pardon.

Scève begins his collection of love poems, or almost so, since this is the second dizain of over four hundred, with this mad turning-toward, as if he had sublimated the gesture of Orpheus and of Laura and Petrarch.[33] What is left is a discursive movement, not a physical one: the turning to glance becomes the apostrophe and then a logical move from the universal to the particular. Perhaps this discursive movement relies for its effectiveness on the sedimentation of physical gestures, as Virgil had so brilliantly demonstrated. The poet-lover maintaining himself to be the exception, the particular case to which attention is turned, is relying on the empathy that, perhaps, *any* turning toward another person produces. In this sense the lover is asking pardon or understanding, as Petrarch himself did at the very beginning of his *Canzoniere*, of the reader, and asking pardon of the beloved.

* * *

In concluding, and with all of these meanings of the lover's *turn* in mind, I propose to jump ahead to one of the most succinct scenes of the meeting of (future) lovers in French early modern literature, the encounter of the very young—and just married—Princess de Clèves with the dashing Monsieur de Nemours, at a ball held at the court of Henri II:

> [C]omme elle dansoit avec M. de Guise, il se fit un assez grand bruit vers la porte de la sale, comme de quelqu'un qui entroit et à qui on faisoit place. Mme de Clèves acheva de danser, et pendant qu'elle cherchoit des yeux quelqu'un qu'elle avoit dessein de prendre, le Roy luy cria de prendre celui qui arrivoit. Elle se tourna et vid un homme qu'elle crut d'abord ne pouvoir estre que M. de Nemours, qui passoit par-dessus quelque siège pour arriver où l'on dansoit.[34]

> [As she was dancing with M. de Guise, there was a loud noise over by the door of the ballroom as of people giving way to someone coming in. Mme de Clèves finished dancing, and while she was looking round to find someone she intended to take as a partner, the King called to her to take the person who had just arrived. She turned [*Elle se tourna*] and saw a man who she felt at once could be no other than M. de Nemours stepping over a seat to make his way to where the dancing was.]

The kinetic elements of this first encounter seem to be dominated by M. de Nemours stepping over a chair, demonstrating perfect mastery of his body and the right amount of *négligence* to impress the court audience, and making a beeline toward the dance floor and the Princess. Indeed, the kinetic detail of Nemours' action is striking.[35] However, his movement and our kinesic understanding of that movement, are preceded by and made possible by the *turn* of the Princess toward him. Indeed, the turning of the Princess is followed immediately by her perception of someone who *could be no other than M. de Nemours* (*ne pouvoir estre que M. de Nemours*): the turn is the indicating of the utterly particular. Turning and seeing are so close to each other that they are practically simultaneous: the body has pre-enacted what the visual perception will only confirm. All of the collected meanings of the turn can operate here, once again: it is lovers meeting, lovers are possessed by a madness, any spectator at the court and any reader can empathize with those lovers, and the lovers are doomed. We imitate that turn to the lover who comes to us through the assembled court, and cannot *not* know what this will mean, because of what it has meant. Our kinesic intelligence allows us to treat the following narrative as a deductive process, something that is implied by the very first movement of the Princess de Clèves.[36]

One can easily argue that all of what I have traced in these texts could be, and indeed was, assembled through the combined forces of historical hermeneutics, using commentaries, semantic analysis through context, of rhetoric (catachresis, apostrophe, irony, *evidentia*, etc.), of the understanding that successive poets in history express of a recurring scenario, and even philosophical and legal treatments of equity. However, the physical gesture of turning provides the key to an historical ecology, or what I have called sedimentation over time, of the tragedy of lovers' "madness." It allows us as perceivers of the scenario to be moved by empathy, quite literally, as it enacts an argument for exception, for "equity," that all of us can re-enact. This relation of *all* readers and perceivers to what is *unique*, utterly particular, is often expressed in poetry in ways that go beyond representation of kinesis, through the—often abrupt—transition from statements claiming general validity to statements emphasizing the singularity or particularity of an event or an affect. In this sense the *turn* is the physical substratum of the dialectical or logical move from universal to particular, in the manner of a catachresis, and, I would argue, this catachresis functions over time, as an enactment and a recalling that is particularly compelling in the European tradition of love. The concept of kinesic intelligence allows us as interpreters of literature to connect the dots, as it were. It allows us to understand how love lyric and ethics can be integrated, as an expression of and a response to a physical intentional scenario that perhaps only a poet such as Virgil can convey to us with such meaning *and* pre-rational force.

Notes

1. Or, as one neuroscientist would say, "unity-in-love" (Semir Zeki), or the "excitatory" (balanced, however, by the "inhibitory" or "aversive," according to Patrick Colm Hogan); see Hogan, "What Literature Teaches Us About Emotion: Synthesizing Affective Science and Literary Study," in *The Oxford Handbook to Cognitive Literary Studies*, ed. Lisa Zunshine (Oxford: Oxford University Press, 2015), 273–90.
2. In the sense that movement is an expression of the body's animation, possessing a soul. In the early modern period one finds frequently the expression "il était sans mouvement et sans vie" ["he was without movement and life,"] (unless noted otherwise, all translations my own) (Jean-Pierre Camus); when Montaigne describes himself as dead, following his fall from his horse, he says of himself lying there: "moi … n'ayant ny mouvement ny sentiment" ["me … having no … movement or sensation"]; *Les Essais*, ed. Pierre Villey and Verdun-L. Saulnier (Paris: Presses universitaires de France, 1965) II.6, 373; *The Complete Essays*, trans. M.A. Screech (London: Penguin, 1987), 419. "Mouvement" comes before "vie" and before "sentiment." On signs of life as a special case of eliciting kinesic intelligence, see Raphael Lyne in this volume.
3. I prefer the Virgilian version of Orpheus's *katábasis* to Ovid's, because Virgil is the first in the Orphic tradition to impart to the poet the role of tragic lover, and this scene is more intensely affecting than Ovid's revision, which allows Eurydice only a faint "Vale" in response to her husband's turning toward her. Also, it is distinctly "empathetic," to use Brooks Otis' term, in relation to the Aristaeus portions of the fourth *Georgic*. See Charles Segal, *Orpheus: The Myth of the Poet* (Baltimore: Johns Hopkins University Press, 1989), 40. Already Cristoforo Landino remarked, on Eurydice's short speech (which is absent from Ovid): "oratio vehementer pathetica. Nam & suum vehementer exprimit dolorem. Demonstrat enim eo devenisse amantes, ut culpa illius qui nihil minus quam hoc voluisset infoelicissimo, & aeterno dissidio separentur" ["a vehemently pathetic speech. For she expresses vehemently her pain. She demonstrates indeed to him that the lovers had descended to this, that through the fault of him who wanted nothing less than this, they would be separated by a terrible and eternal divide"]; see *Aeneis Virgiliana cum Servii Honorati grammatici huberrimis commentariis* (Lyon: Jean Crespin, 1529), 264.
4. Trans. H. Rushton Fairclough (Cambridge, MA: Harvard University Press, rev. ed. 1999). I have modified the translation to make it more literal.
5. My focus on the gestures means that all the resonances of the myth in these lines cannot be dealt with: the Orpheus legend and the Orphic ritual tradition are much too varied and rich. For a summary overview of the myth of

Orpheus and its history up to contemporary times, see Sergio Ferrarese, *Sulle tracce di Orfeo: storia di un mito* (Pisa: ETS, 2010); also, for a florilegium of texts recounting the myth, Marina Di Simone, *Amore e morte in uno sguardo: Il mito di Orfeo e Euridice tra passato e presente* (Florence: Libri Liberi, 2003). I will also refrain from alluding to significant later readings or versions of this scene, such as we find in Rilke or in Blanchot, which are rewritings or allegories little interested in the articulation of the classical text itself. I will also not consider the lines within the larger context of the epyllion.

6. See Kathryn Banks' essay on the "revival" of embodied meanings, in this volume.
7. Or, as Kathryn Banks and Timothy Chesters formulate it, a "complex cognitive ecology" (Introduction).
8. As Neil Kenny helpfully pointed out during our discussion. My thanks to Jan Miernowski for his comments on this essay, as well. On syntax and kinesis, see Terence Cave in this volume.
9. Virgil insists, then, that this law is given by Proserpina (and the "tyrant" in l. 492 seems to refer to Pluto), not by Orpheus himself. Servius, rather ungenerously, characterizes Orpheus's transgression as one against a law he "gave himself": "Nam respiciendo commisit in legem sibi datam" ["For looking back he violated the law he had given himself"] see *Aeneis Virgiliana*, 264.
10. "Furiosus nullum negotium gerere potest, quia non intellegit, quid agit" ["The demented person cannot conduct any business, for he does not understand what he is doing"]; *Institutes* 3.19.8; ed. Paul Krueger, trans. Peter Birks and Grant McLeod (Ithaca: Cornell University Press, 1987). Furthermore, "furiosi [testamentum facere non possunt], quia mente carent" ["Demented persons cannot make a testament, for they are deficient in mind"] (2.12.1). Orpheus' *dementia* thus takes on a specific juridical significance, and reinforces reasons to exercise clemency.
11. See Guillemette Bolens: "Perceptual simulations are dynamic perceptual acts [corresponding to intentions to produce meaning, rather than to defined, isolatable, and fixed mental products]"; *The Style of Gestures: Embodiment and Cognition in Literary Narrative* (Baltimore: Johns Hopkins University Press, 2012), 6 [translation completed to reflect French original].
12. *L'Opere di Virgilio Mantoano, cioè, la Bucolica, la Georgica, e l'Eneide, commentate in lingua volgare toscana da Giovanni Fabrini da Fighine, Carlo Malatesta da Rimene, & Filippo Venuti da Cortona* (Venice: I Sessa, 1615), f. 99[r], my trans. following. Which is a version of Cristoforo Landino's comment: "Ignoscenda,] nam si cognosceremus quam misere cupiant amantes visere rem amatam, & quam vehemens sit haec perturbatio in hac re iudicaremus illis huiuscemodi erratum condonandum. Sed manes propter illorum

crudelitatem nullam noverunt humanitatem" [["Ignoscenda,] for if we knew how miserably lovers desire to see the one loved, and how violent this trouble is, we would judge in this matter to forgive them this kind of error"]; *Aeneis Virgiliana*, 264. The "paraphrase" of Nicolas Grimald expands upon Landino: "Quis enim intelligens quam misere cupiant amantes rem amatam aspicere, quamque vehemens sit haec perturbatio, non existimet huiusmodi erratum condonandum? Sed profecto Dii manes, propter eorum innatam crudelitatem nulla moventur humanitate ad quamlibet lenem culpam remittendam. At in quo peccatum est.? cum[?] quae tenuit eum dementia?" ["Who indeed understanding how wretchedly lovers desire to look at their beloved, and how violent this trouble is, would he not think this kind of error to be pardoned? But certainly the spirits of the god, because of their natural cruelty, are moved by no humanity to pardon any slight fault. And where is the sin? Since a dementia possessed him?"]; *In P. V. Maronis quatuor libros Georgicorum in oratione soluta Paraphrasis*, London, George Bishop & Radulphus Newbery, 1591, f. 99[v].

13. The same terms are used in the Italian translation and amplification of Orpheus's forgetfulness of Proserpina's law (*immemor*): "Scordato oime, de l'aspra legge iniqua" ["Forgotten, alas, the harsh inequitable law"]; *L'Opere di Vergilio Cioè la Bucolica, la Georgica, & l'Eneida, Nuovamente da Diversi Eccellentissimi auttori tradotte in versi sciolti, Et con ogni diligentia raccolte da M. Lodovico Domenichi* (Florence: Giunti, 1556), f. 91[v]. A "legge iniqua" calls for its opposite, a judgment of equity. "Aspra" and "iniqua" are two epithets commonly given to death.
14. Whereas Virgil accumulates juridical elements that seem to solicit clemency on behalf of Orpheus, Ovid arguably refuses to do so, explaining the poet's violation of Proserpina's "law" by his fear that his wife might be failing to follow him, and by his longing to see her: "hic, ne deficeret, metuens avidusque videndi / flexit amans oculos" ["he, afraid that she might fail him, eager for the sight of her, turned back his longing eyes"]; *Metamorphoses*, ed. and trans. Frank Justus Miller (Cambridge, MA; Harvard University Press, 1984) X.56–7. Virgil insists on the cruel nature of the "tyrant" who imposed a condition upon her return, whereas Ovid only uses the term "cruel" after the episode, when he reports that Orpheus complained that the gods were cruel: "esse deos Erebi crudeles questus" ["complaining that the gods of Erebus were cruel"], X.76). Despite his wife's tacit acceptance of her husband's error, he remains a responsible partner in the pact with Proserpina, unlike the Orpheus of Virgil, overcome with a *furor* that makes him incapable of fulfilling (and even entering into) a legal contract.
15. On apostrophe and the lyric, see most recently Jonathan Culler, *Theory of the Lyric* (Cambridge, MA: Harvard University Press, 2015), 211–43. Culler is most interested in apostrophe to things not normally addressed,

and in its emphasis on the present moment (226), a feature of lyric address that heightens the empathetic value of the scene in Virgil.

16. "[I]ncautum è l'epiteto dell'innamorato, perche non è cosa alcuna tanto propria agli innamorati, quanto essere poco accorti, & imprudenti: dice dementia, pazzia, l'esser fuor di sentimento, perche la forza d'amore non è altro, che pazzia" ["'Incautum' is the epithet of the person in love, because there is nothing as appropriate to persons in love, as being little aware and imprudent; he says 'dementia', madness, being out of your senses, since the force of love is none other than madness"] (ibid.). Landino points to the child-like nature of those afflicted by love: "vis amoris dementia est., incautum, nihil tam proprium amanti, unum pueris equiparatur" ["the force of love is madness, careless, nothing is as specific to the lover, one that he shares with the child"]; *Aeneis Virgiliana*, 264. The paronomasia *amans—amens* occurs frequently in the commentary: e.g., Badius Ascensius: "sunt enim amantes ceci & amentes fere" ["indeed, lovers are blind and almost mad"]; ibid.
17. This distinguishes Orpheus and his love for Eurydice from Aristaeus' bees, from their need to merely reproduce and hence their lack of human *amor*, as Segal points out (*Orpheus*, 47).
18. In the Ovidian version, the passive and active forms of *prendere*, in his formulation *prendique et prendere certans* ["and striving to be taken and to take," my trans.] (X.58), similarly underline the (wished-for) reciprocity of gesture uniting the couple.
19. There are many instances in Cicero, and see also Virgil, *Georgics* I.59: "Eliadum palmas Epiros equarum" ["Epiros [gave us] the Olympian victories of her mares"]. A well-known second century painting of the Orpheus-Eurydice episode, taken from a villa in Ostia, and presently in the Vatican museum, shows Eurydice holding her right arm toward her husband, but not stretching her hand; instead, she is presenting him her palm, as if to literalize that Virgilian synecdoche. The image can be seen at: http://www.ostia-antica.org/dict/plnec/plnec.htm (consulted 4 October 2016).
20. All quotations from the *Canzoniere* are taken from the ed. by Marco Santagata (Milan: Mondadori, rev. ed. 2004). English trans. from *Petrarch's Lyric Poems: The Rime sparse and Other Lyrics*, trans. and ed. Robert M. Durling (Cambridge, MA: Harvard University Press, 1976). For related brief analyses of this poem, and Maurice Scève's second dizain of his *Délie*, see my *Lyric in the Renaissance: From Petrarch to Montaigne* (Cambridge: Cambridge University Press, 2015), 151–2 and 154–5; I look at the specifically Petrarchan heritage (not the resonance of Virgil) in Scève's poem in "Legacies of *Rime Sparse* 267 (Petrarch, Ronsard, Scève)," in *Legacies of Petrarch*, ed. Ernesto Livorni, Jelena Todorovic (forthcoming).

21. Which is a movement tying lyric to epic (and as such deserves more attention than I give it here); see Thomas M. Greene, *The Descent from Heaven: A Study in Epic Continuity* (New Haven: Yale University Press, 1963), a study predating cognitive approaches to literature.
22. Commentators note this bursting-forth of emotion, initiating the list of her qualities. Bembo comments: "Comincia adunque piangendo, & dice Oime il bel viso…" ["He begins thus by crying, and says 'Oime il bel viso'…"]; *Il Petrarca con dichiarationi non piu stampate. Insieme con alcune belle Annotationi, tratte dalle dottissime Prose di Monsignor Bembo* (Venice: Nicolò Bevilacqua, 1568), 257; Francesco Filelfo: "dolendosi crida oime bel viso" ["lamenting he cries out 'oime il bel viso'"] and Antonio da Tempo: "In questo sonetto piange el poeta le belleze de la sua donna" ["In this sonnet the poet laments the beauties of his lady"]; *Petrarcha con doi commenti sopra li sonetti et canzone. El primo del ingeniosissimo misser Francesco Philelpho. L'altro del sapientissimo Antonio da Tempo novamente addito* (Venice: Bernardinus Stagninus, 1508), f. 92^{v}.
23. On the distinction between a limited question and an unlimited one, see, although the source is not, perhaps, known to Petrarch himself, the summary in Quintilian, *Institutio oratoria*, III.5.5–7.
24. In defending the poet Archia, Cicero admits that his own oratory is nourished by the reading of poetry (*Pro Archia*, exordium), and that other endeavours are limited in time, in age and in place, whereas poetry belongs to all times and ages and places (vii.16).
25. See, especially for later medieval readers, Quintilian, *Institutio oratoria*, IX.2.38.
26. See Castelvetro's commentary: "Rivolge il parlare all'anima sola, che piu non ha il corpo con seco…" ["He turns his speech to the soul alone, which no longer has the body with it"]; *Le Rime del Petrarca brevemente sposte per Lodovico Castelvetro* (Basel: Pietro de Sedabonis, 1582), Parte seconda, 1.
27. The apostrophe to the soul recalls Laura's evocation as "humile in tanta gloria" ["humble in such glory"] (126, l. 44), and it is no less ambiguous: whereas Laura's bestowing of hope on the poet, in the concluding tercet, conforms to the qualities of the Virgin redeeming the original sin of Eve, the desire that she also provokes in the poet-lover runs counter to the identification of Laura and Mary. The political connotations are also deeply problematic in these two lines, and the commentary tradition is justifiably divided on their meaning.
28. Petrarch mostly addresses Laura in the second-person plural: e.g. "son già roco,/donna, mercé chiamando, et voi non cale […] da voi sola procede … il sole e 'l foco…" ["I am already hoarse, Lady, with calling for mercy, and you do not care […] from you alone come forth the sun and the fire"], 133, ll. 3–4, 8), but sometimes not: "Tu sola mi piaci" ["You alone please me"] (205, l. 8).

29. *Le Rime* ..., Parte seconda, 1. My translation. In the note to l. 1 Castelvetro uses similar language of Laura's attributes as "goods": "Altrove annovera i beni in Laura..." ["Elsewhere he lists the goods in Laura..."]; ibid.
30. Vellutello used the same expression, but locating the apostrophe at the beginning of the first tercet: "E volgendo a lei il parlare dice, che quantunque ella sia morta, convenirli però anchora per lei ardere, & in lei respirare" ["And turning to her his speech, he says that even though she is dead, it is still appropriate for him to burn for her and to breathe by her"]; *Il Petrarcha con l'espositione d'Alessandro Vellutello e con piu utili cose in diversi luoghi di quella novissimamente da lui aggiunte* (Vinegia; Bartolomeo Zanetti Casterzagense, 1538), f. 99[r].
31. Death can be characterized, among others, by the following epithets, according to Ravisius Textor: *frigida, rigida, acerba, nigra, crudelis, indomita, saeva, dura, violenta, cruenta, squallida, misera, gelida, turpis, aspera, cruda, iniqua, terribilis, tristis, impia* ["cold, rigid, bitter, black, cruel, unconquered, vicious, hard, violent, bloody, harsh, miserable, icy, hideous, harsh, savage, inequitable, terrifying, sad, impious"]; cited in his *Epitheta Ioannis Ravisii Textoris Nivernensis* ... (Rouen: Romanus de Beauvais, 1612), f. 310[r]–311[r]. But it is also "æqua" ["equal"], since it affects everyone.
32. Dizain 2, ed. Eugène Parturier (Paris: Nizet, 5th ed. 1987), 6; my trans.
33. In his 1552 *Amours*, Pierre de Ronsard imitates Scève's second *dizain* (and Petrarch as well), in the *second* sonnet: "Tout ce qu'Amour avarement couvoit/De beau, de chaste, & d'honneur sous ses aeles,/Emmïélla les graces immortelles/De son bel œil, qui les dieus émouvoit/Du ciel à peine elle étoit descendue,/Quand je la vi, quand mon ame éperdue/En devint folle" ["Everything that Love greedily hatched, everything beautiful, chaste and honourable, under its wings, she sweetened the immortal graces with her beautiful eye, which moved the gods. Hardly had she descended from the sky when I saw her, when my bewildered soul went mad for her"]; ed. André Gendre (Paris: Libraire générale française, 1993) 82, l. 5–11). Similar *katábasis*, this time explicit, similar contrast between all goods and only me, similar perception of the beloved by the soul, and the same result: amorous frenzy. See Timothy Chesters' commentary on the first dizain of the *Délie*, in this volume.
34. Madame de Lafayette, *La Princesse de Clèves*, in *Romanciers du XVIIe siècle*, ed. Antoine Adam (Paris: Gallimard, 1958), 1126. The translation is by Terence Cave, quoted in his *Thinking with Literature: Towards a Cognitive Criticism* (Oxford: Oxford University Press, 2016, 115). On the inaugural scene of exchanged glances, see Jean Rousset, *Leurs yeux se rencontrèrent* (Paris: José Corti, 1981); this scene does not reproduce the archetypal model, preferring, as Cave rightly points out, sound and physical movement to mere visual encounter.

35. See the analysis by Cave, *Thinking with Literature*, 114–20, who limits himself to the actions of Nemours.
36. However, our kinaesthetic knowledge of her movement, and the history of this particular movement, set us up for the reversal that is the key to the novel. The Princess de Clèves is quite literally *inimitable*, for she alone, of all lovers from Orpheus and Eurydice to Petrarch and Laura and so many others, she alone refuses to participate in the scenario that her turning to Nemours has made seemingly inevitable.

Bibliography

Bolens, Guillemette. *The Style of Gestures: Embodiment and Cognition in Literary Narrative*. Baltimore: Johns Hopkins University Press, 2012.

Cave, Terence. *Thinking with Literature: Towards a Cognitive Criticism*. Oxford: Oxford University Press, 2016.

Culler, Jonathan. *Theory of the Lyric*. Cambridge, MA: Harvard University Press, 2015.

Di Simone, Marina. *Amore e morte in uno sguardo: Il mito di Orfeo e Euridice tra passato e presente*. Florence: Libri Liberi, 2003.

Ferrarese, Sergio. *Sulle tracce di Orfeo: storia di un mito*. Pisa: ETS, 2010.

Greene, Thomas M. *The Descent from Heaven: A Study in Epic Continuity*. New Haven: Yale University Press, 1963.

Hogan, Patrick Colm. What Literature Teaches Us About Emotion: Synthesizing Affective Science and Literary Study. In *The Oxford Handbook to Cognitive Literary Studies*, edited by Lisa Zunshine, 273–90. Oxford: Oxford University Press, 2015.

Justinian. *Institutes*. Edited by Paul Krueger, translated by Peter Birks and Grant McLeod. Ithaca: Cornell University Press, 1987.

Lafayette, Madame de. *La Princesse de Clèves*, in *Romanciers du XVIIe siècle*, edited by Antoine Adam. Paris: Gallimard, 1958.

Landino, Cristoforo. *Aeneis Virgiliana cum Servii Honorati grammatici huberrimis commentariis*. Lyon: Jean Crespin, 1529.

Langer, Ullrich. *Lyric in the Renaissance: From Petrarch to Montaigne*. Cambridge: Cambridge University Press, 2015.

———. Legacies of *Rime Sparse* 267 (Petrarch, Ronsard, Scève). In *Legacies of Petrarch*, edited by Ernesto Livorni and Jelena Todorovic (forthcoming).

Montaigne, Michel de. *Les Essais*. Edited by Pierre Villey and Verdun-L. Saulnier. Paris: Presses universitaires de France, 1965.

Ovid. *Metamorphoses: Books 9–15*. Translated by Frank Justus Miller, 2nd ed. Cambridge, MA: Harvard University Press, 1984.

Petrarch, Francis. *Petrarcha con doi commenti sopra li sonetti et canzone. El primo del ingeniosissimo misser Francesco Philelpho. L'altro del sapientissimo Antonio da Tempo novamente addito...* Venice: Bernardinus Stagninus, 1508.

———. *Il Petrarcha con l'espositione d'Alessandro Vellutello e con piu utili cose in diversi luoghi di quella novissimamente da lui aggiunte.* Vinegia: Bartolomeo Zanetti Casterzagense, 1538.

———. *Il Petrarca con dichiarationi non piu stampate. Insieme con alcune belle Annotationi, tratte dalle dottissime Prose di Monsignor Bembo...* Venice: Nicolò Bevilacqua, 1568.

———. *Le Rime del Petrarca brevemente sposte per Lodovico Castelvetro.* Basel: Pietro de Sedabonis, 1582.

———. *Petrarch's Lyric Poems: The Rime Sparse and Other Lyrics.* Edited and translated by Robert M. Durling. Cambridge, MA: Harvard University Press, 1976.

———. *Canzoniere.* Edited by Marco Santagata. 2nd ed. Milan: Mondadori, 2004.

Ronsard, Pierre de. *Les Amours et les Folastries (1552–1560).* Edited by André Gendre. Paris: Libraire générale française, 1993.

Rousset, Jean. *Leurs yeux se rencontrèrent.* Paris: José Corti, 1981.

Scève, Maurice. *Delie, object de plus haulte vertu.* Edited by Eugène Parturier. 5th ed. Paris: Nizet, 1987.

Segal, Charles. *Orpheus: The Myth of the Poet.* Baltimore: Johns Hopkins University Press, 1989.

Textor, Ravisius (Jean Tixier de Ravisi). *Epitheta Ioannis Ravisii Textoris Nivernensis.* Rouen: Romanus de Beauvais, 1612.

Virgil. *Aeneis Virgiliana cum Servii Honorati grammatici huberrimis commentariis.* Lyon: Jean Crespin, 1529.

———. *L'Opere di Vergilio Cioè la Bucolica, la Georgica, & l'Eneida, Nuovamente da Diversi Eccellentissimi auttori tradotte in versi sciolti, Et con ogni diligentia raccolte da M. Lodovico Domenichi.* Florence: Giunti, 1556.

———. *In P. V. Maronis quatuor libros Georgicorum in oratione soluta Paraphrasis.* London: George Bishop & Radulphus Newbery, 1591.

———. *L'Opere di Virgilio Mantoano, cioè, la Bucolica, la Georgica, e l'Eneide, commentate in lingua volgare toscana da Giovanni Fabrini da Fighine, Carlo Malatesta da Rimene, & Filippo Venuti da Cortona.* Venice: I Sessa, 1615.

———. *Georgics.* Translated by H. Rushton Fairclough. Rev ed. Cambridge, MA: Harvard University Press, 2006.

CHAPTER 4

Scève's Denominal Verbs

Timothy Chesters

In the final pages of Pontus de Tyard's Neoplatonic dialogue *Solitaire premier* (1552), the discussion between the Solitaire and his Muse Pasithée turns to obscurity in poetry. What, Pasithée asks the Solitaire, do you and your poet friends say to those who complain that by "si estranges façons de parler" ("such strange ways of speaking") your verse so obscures your thought that common folk can no longer recognize their own tongue?[1] Accusations of verbal obscurantism were topical in the early 1550s. Tyard being a minor member of the "Brigade" (the circle of poets later known as the Pléiade), Pasithée may have in mind the unapologetically elitist renewal of the French language promoted in Joachim Du Bellay's *Deffence et illustration de la langue françoise* (1549) and practised in Pierre de Ronsard's *Odes* (1550).[2] But Tyard also had connections to the earlier generation of Lyonnais poets grouped around the notoriously obscure Maurice Scève, and it is in recalling the Solitaire's response to one reader of Scève's *Délie* (1544) that, by way of a brief reminiscence, a smiling Pasithée answers her own question:

T. Chesters (✉)
Clare College, Cambridge, UK

K. Banks, T. Chesters (eds.), *Movement in Renaissance Literature*, Cognitive Studies in Literature and Performance,
https://doi.org/10.1007/978-3-319-69200-5_4

> Vous souvient-il point [...] de celuy qui un jour arrivant icy, me trouva une Delie en main: et de quelle grace, l'ayant prinse et encor non leu le second vers entier, il se rida le front et la jetta sus la table à demy courroucé?—Oh, si fais déa (respondy-je) et ay bien memoire qu'entre autres choses, quand je le vy autant nouveau et incapable d'entendre la raison, que les doctes vers du Seigneur Maurice Scæve [...] je luy respondis, qu'aussi se soucioit bien peu le Seigneur Maurice que sa Delie fust veuë, ny maniée des veaux.[3]

> [Do you not remember that gentleman who, turning up here one day, found me reading a copy of *Délie*, and how gracefully he took it up and, having not got to the end of the second line, frowned and threw the book down on the table half in anger?—Oh, yes indeed I do (I replied) and remember clearly, among other things, that when I saw him as novice-like and little capable of understanding reason as the learned verses of Monsieur Maurice Scève [...] I replied that Monsieur Maurice cared very little to see his Delie seen and handled by dolts.]

"Il se rida le front et la jetta sur la table": though here the butt of the Tyard's laughter, the unnamed reader's gesture sums up a widespread exasperation with the *Délie*, Scève's sequence of 449 ten-line epigrams or *dizains*, fusing Petrarchan motifs, Neoplatonic mysticism and the recent vogue for emblems. Notable for his syntactical compression and ellipses, the writer whom Ferdinand Brunetière later condemned as a "poète illisible" ["unreadable poet"] was already reproached for his obscurity in his own lifetime, prompting friends like Tyard to come to his defence.[4] In literary historical terms, it was not until well after poetic difficulty was made newly fashionable by Brunetière's late nineteenth-century contemporaries, notably Verlaine and Mallarmé, that readers found the patience to take up the *Délie* again.

This essay offers a new approach to some of Scève's "estranges façons de parler" by treating these as instances of radical *underspecification*. Strictly speaking that term belongs to the vocabulary of Gricean pragmatics, where it describes the basic fact that most of what we say underspecifies—or underdetermines—the content of what we actually mean.[5] Speakers of a language do not simply encode their meaning in an utterance for others to decipher using an identical copy of the code. Rather the sounds they utter, and the conceptual information these sounds encode, offer only an initial cue or prompt—a jumping-off point—from which the hearer must "fill out" the speaker's meaning inferentially. The perspective from pragmatics has strongly influenced what follows, where references to "underspecification" are intended in just this sense. But a similar phenomenon can also be considered a component of kinesis. According to the approach adopted in this volume, the information carried by a sensorimotor prompt—the kinaesthetic "echo" of another's motion, gesture or posture—never arrives in our cognitive apparatus as a fully formed apprehension of the other's mental states. Here too the information is underspecified; sensorimotor resonance offers an incomplete if powerful grasp of the other's inner life—whether of their "expressive direction," in Guillemette Bolens's phrase, or simply the biological fact that "someone is at home."[6] Determining the precise expressive content of a particular movement, in all its tangled imbrication with so called higher-order information (cultural knowledge, for example), is a difficult task. It requires our kinesic intelligence—a know-how that poetry calls upon with special urgency, and Scève's poems more than most.

***

One feature of Scève's *Délie* has been singled out as a special barrier to comprehension: its neologisms.[7] The latter years of Scève's life (he died in 1564) was a heyday of lexical renewal in France, led by the younger Pléiade poets, who tended to admire him.[8] Guillaume des Autelz, for instance, praises Scève's "magnificence de mots innovez et translatez" ("magnificence of his newly coined and imported words").[9] But others were less glowing. Thomas Sébillet defends Scève against a number of unnamed critics who reproach him for his new words, "sans lesquelz toutesfois l'enargie des choses contenues cellee & moins exprimee, eut fait ignorer bonne part de la conception de l'autheur" ("The roughness of many new words, without which, however, the vividness [*energia*] of its content being hidden within and less explicit, a good deal of the author's conception would have remained unknown").[10] The reference to *energia*, or vividness, seems a striking vindication of Scève's novelties, and yet even Sébillet concedes that often the author's thought remains inaccessible.[11] The late sixteenth-century historian Étienne Pasquier is not so equivocal. On first reading Scève he recalls struggling with "un sens si ténébreux que, le lisant, je disois estre très content de ne l'entendre, puisqu'il ne vouloit estre entendu" ["A meaning so obscure that, reading him, I would say that I was very glad not to understand him, since he did not wish to be understood"].[12] Pasquier was no "veau," but his impatience echoes that of the anonymous reader evoked by Tyard (as well as the Solitaire's response to it). For Pasquier, Scève's indifference to his reader wilfully violates what modern pragmatics terms the "co-operative principle" supposed to subtend all human communication.[13] Although cultivating a certain measure of obscurity was second nature to anyone schooled in the allegorical tradition (of which emblems were a part), for many the *Délie* had overstepped the mark.

Of particular interest to Scève's modern commentators has been the verbal quirk that early modern rhetoricians once called *anthimeria*, and modern lexicology now terms "conversion" or "functional shift": instances where a word of one grammatical class (verbs, nouns, adjectives, etc.) is transposed into another.[14] Particular attention has been paid to his frequently obscure use of substantivized infinitives, for example:

Au receuoir l'aigu de tes esclairs
Tu m'offuscas & sens, & cognoissance [...][15]

[At the receiving the sharp point of your flashes
You assaulted my senses and consciousness]

D80

À l'embrunir des heures tenebreuses [...]
[At the browning of the dark hours]

D126

Motivated in part by their prestige in Greek, Du Bellay would enthusiastically approve of such forms in French: "use donc hardiment de l'infinitif pour le nom" ["make bold use of the infinitive for the noun"], he urges in the *Deffence*, citing as examples "*l'aller, le chanter, le vivre, le mourir*" before further recommending the use of substantivized adjectives (*le liquide des eaux, le vide de l'air, le frais des ombres*), and adverbialized nouns (*ils combattent obstinés*, for *obstinément*).[16] The need for concision imposed by Scève's *dizains* makes instances of conversion especially frequent across his *Délie*, often causing the reader to hesitate or stumble.[17]

One subtype of Scève's functional shifts has been somewhat overlooked so far, namely denominal verbs: that is, where new verbs are formed from nouns. Readers of the *Délie* do not have to wait long for an example. Returning to Pasithée's story, we recall that it was precisely mid-way through the second line of that text that her visitor loses patience: "ayant non leu *le second vers entier*, il se rida le front et la jetta sus la table" (my emphasis). Turning to the opening *dizain* of the sequence, we see that it begins as follows:

L'Œil trop ardent en mes ieunes erreurs
Girouettoit, mal cault, à l'impourueue [...]

D1, 1–2 (my emphasis)

[The too ardent eye of my youthful errors *weather-vaned*, heedless and at random...]

Pasithée's reference to "le second vers" might merely be read as throwaway or approximate: that is, she may simply mean that "he had barely begun reading when... ." But possibly she is being more precise: perhaps the new-fangled verb *girouetter* was what put her visitor in a temper.

Certainly, it has not been sufficiently remarked how peculiar this opening might have sounded to Scève's contemporaries. In line 1 they would naturally have recognized, in the allusion to Petrarch's "primo giovenile errore," what was fast becoming the signature flourish of the newly acclimatized Petrarchan mode in France; four years later, in 1548, Tyard himself would dedicate to Scève his own *Erreurs amoureuses*, with its similar opening reference to "les erreurs de ma jeunesse vaine" ["the errors of my vain youth"]. In Scève's poem, though, the enjambement into line 2 immediately propels them into new territory. Formed from the noun "girouette" (sometimes "gyrouet")—a weather-vane—which itself had only entered French in the early years of the sixteenth-century, the verb *girouetter* appears to have been Scève's own invention. Not for the last time in the *Délie*, a poem sets out on a familiar—even over-familiar—path only to embark on a sudden leftward swerve.

The shock value of Scève's denominal verbs deserves greater attention. One reason for their neglect so far may be that French denominals are less straightforward examples of functional shift than their English counterparts. In French, denominals are usually formed by the addition of [e] to a nominal stem (*balai➔balayer*, *brosse➔brosser*, *beurre➔beurrer*); only in certain parts of the present tense are these indistinguishable from the parent noun ("passe-moi la brosse"/"brosse-moi les cheveux"). Although English can do this too—think of the suffix *-ize* in *demonize*, for instance—it is additionally able to form "purer" instances, where in the infinitive form the noun is left morphologically untouched (*bottle*➔ *bottle*).[18] English instances are also far commoner, especially in verse. Milton and especially Shakespeare use them frequently:

And I come *coffin'd* home. (*Corialanus* 5.1)
It out-*Herods* Herod. (*Hamlet* 5.1)
Petruchio is *Kated*. (*Taming of the Shrew* 3.2)
[...] the hearts/That *spanieled* me at heels. (*Antony and Cleopatra* 4.12)
sea-monsters *tempest* the ocean. (*Paradise Lost* 7.412)

Following the loss of inflectional endings during the early Middle Ages, word-class conversion had become by Shakespeare's time a valuable source of new words and meanings; it may be thanks to him that denominal verb formation in particular has come to be regarded as a distinctively English mode of linguistic creativity.[19] By contrast, French denominals lack this cultural prestige. They are notably absent, for instance, from Louis Guilbert's influential 1975 study of conversion and neologism, *La Créativité lexicale*.[20]

Be that as it may, sixteenth-century French poets and lexicographers were certainly alert to the creative potential of such forms. Denominal verbs seem to have been prized for their regional and, especially, archaic flavour. Despite Du Bellay's antipathy to medieval verse forms, he regrets the loss of certain words commonly found among "tous ces vieux romans et poetes françois" ["all those old French romancers and poets"]: he cites in particular the verbs *ajourner* ([of the day] to break) and *anuiter* ([of the night] to fall).[21] Ronsard agrees, urging poets in his *Abrégé de la poétique françoise* (1565) to follow their medieval predecessors in adapting known nouns into exotic new verbs: *verve* into *verver*, *essoine* into *essoiner*, *feu* into *fouer*, *pays* to *payser*.[22] Similar remarks can be found in the *Art poëtique* (1555) of Jacques Peletier du Mans, who confesses his fondness for *encrucher* (to lodge something between the branches of a tree) and *arrocher* (to hurl stones), both local to Le Mans.[23] Henri Estienne provides the fullest sixteenth-century treatment in his *La Precellence de la langue françoise* (1579), where he lists vanished denominals found in the medieval romances: *addenter* (to hit the floor with one's teeth having fallen off a horse), *borgnoyer* (to cast a sidelong glance), *paumoyer un baton* (to handle), *archoyer* (to fire a bow), *enflecher* (to pierce with arrows), *soleiller* (to walk in the sun), *se hérissonner* (to curl up into a ball), and so on.[24] Presumably for Scève too denominal morphology possessed this archaizing flavour, making novel coinages like "girouetter" a striking amalgam of the old and the new.

Around twenty denominal verbs can be found in the *Délie*, many of which were either new or nearly new to French in 1544. They come in two forms. One sub-class is formed with prefixes: *encendrir* (to turn to ashes; D264), *obtenebrer* (to grow dark; D178), *ahontir* (to make ashamed; D166), *apourir* (to make afraid; D166), *s'ajourner* ([of the day] to break; D265). The other follows the pattern of *girouetter* in being forged from nouns denoting objects or animate creatures: for example, *pirouetter* (to pirouette; D137), *se crester* (to crest; D175), *sagetter* (to arrow; D268), *deluger* (to flood; D50), *flocquer* ([of snowfall] to thicken?; D9), *satyriser* (to dance like a satyr?; D104), *chevecher* (to owl?, to wear a bonnet?; D57), and *se paonner* (to peacock; D58, D318). This latter class of denominals is especially relevant for our purposes because in almost all cases readers are invited to infer from them a particular form of *motion*. In the first category mentioned above (*s'ajourner*, *obtenebrer*) motion—whether towards or away—is signalled in the prefix; in the second the verbs appeal instead to the reader's perceptual and kinesic memory of how objects and creatures move. Making sense of Scève's denominal verbs requires us, in varying degrees, to deploy our kinesic intelligence.

Underspecification and Inference

Before coming in more detail to Scève's denominal coinages, it may be helpful to consider this inferential process from a theoretical viewpoint. The one adopted here is that of lexical pragmatics, especially as conducted by the Stanford linguists Eve and Herbert Clark in the 1970s and 1980s and then, in updated form, by Relevance Theorists Deirdre Wilson and Robyn Carston. For linguists working in pragmatics, neologisms in general—and novel denominal verbs in particular—present a paradigmatic case of language users' ability to construe each other's meaning inferentially, that is over and beyond the concepts already available in their pre-existing mental lexicon. From their perspective, it is a feature of almost all linguistic utterances that they are radically underspecified with regard to their semantic content. On this view decoding the semantic content of an utterance is almost always insufficient to grasp a speaker's meaning; rather, speakers and listeners constantly co-operate to infer each other's intentions from underspecified linguistic cues. Innovative uses of language, whose intended meaning has by definition to be worked out "on the fly," are especially revealing of how this process works.

Clark and Clark's influential 1979 paper, "When Nouns Surface as Verbs," analyses a corpus of around 1300 lexicalized denominal verbs in English, as well as some interesting hypotheses regarding the use of novel cases. The authors introduce their discussion by noting our remarkable ability to create and deploy expressions we have never heard before:

> In the right contexts, we readily understand *He enfant terrible'd gracefully* (said of a workshop participant), or *Ruling in the death of Ferrari woman* (newspaper headline referring to a woman whose will stipulated that she be buried in her Ferrari), or *Never ask two China trips to the same dinner party* (cartoon caption referring to people who had taken trips to China)—even though we have never before heard *enfant terrible* used as a verb, *Ferrari woman* used as a compound noun, or *China trips* used as a shorthand expression.[25]

A certain measure of any linguistic creativity can be explained by what Clark and Clark call "rules of composition" (they give the example of *ritualness*, composed of *ritual* and—*ness* according to the ordinary rules of English morphology). And yet, they go on:

> Innovations such as *enfant terrible'd*, *Ferrari woman*, and *China trips* do not appear to be explainable in that way. To decide what they mean on a particular occasion, we must know not only the meanings of their parts, but also something about the time, place, and circumstances in which they are uttered.[26]

This mysterious ability to generate novel meanings instantaneously, as the particular occasion demands, is what their study sets out to explain.

Clark and Clark begin by assuming that ordinary denominal verbs should be expected to exhibit some connection to the "parent" noun from which they were historically derived: thus for example "the verb *to bottle* bears some relation, at least diachronically, to its parent noun *bottle*."[27] But the way in which this relation operates is revealed to differ quite considerably from case to case. The authors propose a rough taxonomy of six main categories, excluding metaphorical instances (*the two defenders sandwiched the striker*, *she just parrotted the lesson*, etc.). Their schema can be briefly summarized as follows:

1. LOCATUM verbs: *blanket the bed, roof the house, bridge the river, frame the picture, sugar the tea, skin the rabbit.*
2. LOCATION verbs: *ground the planes, shelve the books, kennel the dog, headquarter the troops.*
3. DURATION verbs: *summer in Paris, vacation in Italy, weekend in Scotland, honeymoon in the Canaries.*
4. AGENT verbs: *butcher the cow, referee the game, tutor the boys, champion the cause, father the child, hound the politician, ape the teacher, squirrel away the money, (out)fox the opponent, to clown around.*
5. GOAL verbs: *powder an aspirin, fool the man, outlaw the thief, martyr the woman, scapegoat the immigrants, cuckold his neighbour, group the actors, parade the troops, bundle the clothes, coil the rope, crease the tablecloth, cream the butter.*
6. INSTRUMENT verbs: *to bicycle, telephone, bolt, screw, staple, mop, hoover, hammer a nail, knife a man, torpedo the ship, shield the child, ladle the soup, shovel the dirt.*

Clark and Clark's typology concludes with several "miscellaneous" sub-categories not covered by these six: these include meals (*lunch, breakfast, feast*), crops (*blackberry in the woods, whale, fish, crab, shrimp*), elements (*snow, rain, hail*), and parts (*kneecap the businessman, his ball lipped the hole* [in golf]). We should note in passing that French denominals can be similarly categorized: Christophe Bogacki notes the different relations between verbs and parent nouns in *arbitrer* (agent: to act as *arbitre* or umpire), *baver* (goal: to produce *la bave*, or saliva), *baigner* (location: to plunge into a liquid, in a *bain*, or bath), and *scier* (instrument: to use a *scie*, or saw).[28] Bogacki remarks that, as in English, the large majority of French denominals belong to the "instrument" type.

Clark and Clark's taxonomy suggests at first glance that speakers access the meaning of denominal verbs via a finite set of semantic derivations. At the time their paper was published, this view was widely accepted. Clark and Clark cite Hans Marchand's claim that "denominal verbs are verbalized sentences," and so should be regarded simply as "translating" a more extended proposition.[29] On this account the meaning of utterances such as *George shelved the books, Rachel bicycled into town* or *Steven butchered the cow* can be captured by a straightforward paraphrase:

(a) George shelved the books. (location)
(b) George did something to make it come about that the books were on the shelf.

(a) Rachel bicycled into town. (instrument)
(b) Rachel caused it to come about that she was in town by performing the act one would normally expect one to do with a bicycle.

(a) Steven butchered a cow. (agent)
(b) Steven did something to a cow that a butcher would normally do.

But Clark and Clark's analysis presents several difficulties for the "verbalized sentences" view. First they raise the objection that many of the historical origins of common denominal verbs are now obscure: few speakers go back to Captain Boycott (say) or Judge Lynch or writing slates when hearing *boycott the store, lynch the prisoner* or *slate the event*. Second, a number of denominals seem to derive from sentences that do not contain the parent noun. They give the example of *land* and *park*: if these really meant "put onto land" and "put into a park," how could one land on a lake or park in a garage? Third and relatedly, semantic idiosyncrasies can be found in even the most common denominal verbs: why should *land the plane* mean "put down the plane" and *ground the plane* mean "keep down the plane" and not the other way around?

And then there is a further, more far-reaching problem. As the authors readily acknowledge, many denominals do not fit neatly into their proposed categories, or rather fit into several categories at once. For example, Brian can *bottle the wine* (location), but he can also turn up at the restaurant and *bottle his wife's lover* (instrument). Even the same action could be construed in diverse ways. In the phrase *George smokes the pipe*, *smoke* could theoretically be a goal verb: George causes smoke to come out of the pipe. But it could also be regarded as a locatum verb (George extracts smoke from the pipe), or perhaps even an instrument verb, since he is doing what one would do with smoke—namely inhaling and exhaling it. Even when two senses belong to the same category, denominals can throw up unexpected contradictions. In both *Sarah milks the cow* and *Sarah milks the tea*, *milk* is a locatum verb; yet in one Sarah takes milks out and in the other puts milk in. A related difficulty, not explored by Clark and Clark, concerns cross-language divergences in metaphorical denominals (a category deliberately excluded from their study). For example, English *to monkey (around)* and French *singer* ("to imitate") share the same nominal concept: on the semantic derivation model, each would paraphrase a proposition of the kind "to do the kind of thing a monkey does." And yet the meaning of each denominal picks out a very different aspect of the parent noun: playfulness in English, mimicry in French. Such cases further emphasize Clark and Clark's central point: that the path travelled from noun to verb is not always easily retraced.

Clark and Clark's objections to the derivation view will be familiar to any student of pragmatics, namely that denominal verbs are often semantically underspecified—and the number of potential specifications is indefinitely large. This point is made especially clear when the authors return to the question of innovative uses. They give the example of *to teapot*:

> Imagine that Ed and Joe have an odd mutual acquaintance, Max, who occasionally sneaks up and strokes the backs of people's legs with a teapot. One day Ed tells Joe, *Well, this time Max has really gone too far. He tried to teapot a policeman.*

On the semantic derivation account, a language user hearing the phrase *teapot a policeman* would try to derive its meaning with reference to the categories above (instrument, locatum, goal and so on), possibly drawing on the model of verbs such as *to bottle*. Hence *to teapot* could plausibly be understood to mean "bash over the head with a teapot," "offer a teapot to," "turn magically into a teapot": all Joe needs to do is review the six categories and select the right one. But this is not what happens. Joe knows, and Ed knows that Joe knows (and Joe knows that Ed knows that Joe knows) about Max's strange proclivity, and that mutual knowledge alone is enough to arrive at the intended meaning: that is, Max stroked the policeman's leg. Now it is true that in order for Ed to coin the denominal, and for Joe to understand his meaning, both must access—and are some extent constrained by—the content of the encoded concept TEAPOT.[30] *To teapot* cannot be made to mean just anything: real world constraints limit the spectrum of possible actions a teapot permits (its "affordances," to borrow a term from perceptual psychology).[31] Even so, nothing in the encoded concept evoked by *to teapot a policeman* specifies which among those possibilities Ed actually intends. And as the oddness of his usage makes clear, this spectrum is very broad indeed—as broad as the number of possible contexts among which the verb *to teapot* could potentially be uttered.[32]

Joe cannot simply decode Ed's meaning, then; he must infer it on the basis of context together with the knowledge of particulars that he shares with Ed. The resulting concept is not locatable in the two friends' mental repertoire; it is an entirely novel, situation-specific concept fit for the occasion. The importance of context and mutual knowledge is especially clear in metaphorical innovations such as *He enfant terribl'd gracefully out of the room* or *he did a Napoleon*: these differ slightly from the concrete verbs discussed above, in that they invite the listener to infer a likeness of some kind.[33] Denominals formed from proper nouns usually belong to this class. Clark and Clark discuss an example in which Sam tells Helen: *my sister Houdini'd her way out of the locked closet*. Here Sam can only expect Helen to grasp his meaning if he believes that she knows, and that she knows he knows, that Houdini was an escape artist. In the absence of this knowledge, he could not have used the proper noun "Houdini" to mean "escape by trickery." Furthermore, if he believed that Helen knew Houdini's manner of death, or his reputation for exposing the frauds of others, he could also expect her to understand *Joe got Houdini'd in the stomach yesterday* (hit hard without warning) or *I would love to Houdini those ESP experiments* (expose as fraudulent). Indeed, as with *to teapot* one could potentially extend such possible meanings as far as the mutually shared knowledge of facts about Houdini's life allows. Of course, as Clark and Clark point out, in any given instance the number of such meanings is always narrowed to one. But this is achieved not by selecting the most viable option from candidates located in a pre-existing code (one's knowledge of the English language); rather, speakers and listeners co-operate to produce the correct interpretation based on their mutual knowledge and salience in context.

For all the complexity of Clark and Clark's account (justice to which could not be done here) their study conveys above all the fleet-footedness with which language users understand innovative denominal verbs. Despite their novelty, and the difficulty of reliably deriving their meaning from the parent noun (locatum, location, goal, agent, and so on), the cases they discuss pose no special challenge to comprehension. Recent experiments in psycholinguistics report English and French children as young as three years old successfully coining and grasping novel denominal verbs.[34] Deirdre Wilson and Robyn Carston reiterate Clark and Clark's findings in the context of Relevance Theory (a cognitively inflected updating of Gricean pragmatics):

> The speed and apparent ease with which experimental participants understand [...] neologisms suggests that lexical-pragmatic processes apply "on-line" in a flexible, creative and context dependent way.[35]

No rulebook sets out in advance what pattern a new denominal will follow. Instead denominal verbs require and reveal something much more exciting: our capacity to form entirely novel, situation-specific concepts (what Relevance Theorists term "ad-hoc concepts") from moment to moment, as circumstance dictates. That we should grasp these and similar coinages with "ease" testifies to the creative power of all human communicators, not just poets.

Kinesic Prompts

Returning now to the *Délie*, the theoretical emphasis on cognitive ease appears to complicate the standard view of Scève's neologisms. Instead of making them an aspect of his obscurity, the perspective from lexical pragmatics points rather towards the opposite hypothesis: that Scève's denominal verbs should be transparent to his sense. Determining whether or not that hypothesis holds will require a closer look at some selected instances.

All the denominal verbs discussed below are metaphorical coinages, a striking feature of which is their capacity to involve the reader's sense of movement, gesture and posture. They serve as kinesic prompts. Take the example of *se paonner* (to peacock, formed on the noun "paon"), which occurs twice:

> Dont mes pensers guidez par leurs Montioyes,
> *Se paonnoient* tous en leur hault Paradis.
>
> D58, 9–10
>
> [From which my thoughts, guided by their Montjoies,
> All peacocked their way towards lofty Paradise.]
>
> Jà tout haultain *je me paonnois*
> De ce, qu'Amour l'avoit peu inciter [...]
>
> D318, 1–2
>
> [Now I was haughtily peacocking
> Over the idea that, Love could have prompted her [...]]

"Se paonner" in these two cases is evidently being used metaphorically of the speaker and his thoughts—that is, as meaning something like "to act *like* a peacock" or, as one might now say in modern French, "faire le paon." But "like" in what respect? Its flightlessness? The peacock's distinctive call (from which the French "paon" supposedly gets its name)? Neither candidate seems likely. Instead, the presence of "hault" and "haultain," no doubt reinforced by a relatively stable set of symbolic associations, suggests that in each instance the most salient property of the peacock is its prideful appearance. Both occurrences provoke the imagination of a movement: more specifically, of a peacock's strutting and spreading his feathers. The poet is congratulating himself, puffing out his chest, fanning his tail. (In today's informal parlance, some might use another kinesic expression, and say that he's "bigging himself up"). Clearly the precise bundle of imagistic and sensorimotor responses provoked by *se paonner* may differ slightly from those provoked in Scève himself, and likewise from reader to reader. It may include a flash of colour, for instance: in which case we might consider Scève's "pensers" ancestors of Marvell's "green thoughts (in a green shade)." But we should expect enough overlap to suggest that something relatively precise is being transmitted—a sense of movement filled out from an underspecified cue.

The case of *se paonner* falls broadly in line with the suggestion of cognitive ease. The human imagination has little difficulty improvising from the verb *se paonner* the concept of a thought-peacock, or a peacock-thought, strutting around Paradise. It helps, of course, that peacocks and pride are so closely associated in the cultural archive of most early modern Europeans—a form of "mutual knowledge" that Scève could doubtless take for granted. In the *Délie* itself this archive is especially near at hand: emblem XXXIV features an image of a peacock in full display, with the motto "Qui bien se voit orgueil abaisse" ["he who knows himself brings down pride"]. The motto makes the moral dimension of pride especially salient; it also furnishes *se paonner* with a countervailing downward motion ("abaisser") that seems to confirm, by opposition, the essentially kinesic force of the denominal—an upward expansion picked up still more vividly in the closing lines of the following *dizain*: "qui se voit, *l'enflé d'orgueil* abaisse" ["he who understands himself, brings down the one *puffed up with* pride"; D303]. The function of the emblems in the *Délie* is mysterious, and has attracted much discussion. But perhaps a clue may lie in the large number of images that, like this one, seem to hinge on a specific posture or movement. A fuller study might consider how Scève's emblems prime and reinforce the kinesic dimension of his language. This function is most evident in emblems such as "Le Paon," "L'Oyseau au glus" or "La Girouette," each of which furnishes a visual commentary on a corresponding denominal verb (*se paonner*, *dégluer*, *girouetter*). But even where this is not the case, Scève's emblems might still serve to make salient particularly precise forms of movement, setting off patterns of kinesic echo or anticipation across the *Délie* as a whole.[36]

In the case of other denominal verbs the inferential process is less straightforward, however. A notorious instance is the word *chevecher* (D57). Scève is complaining that, as in a game of "Mousche" (l.1) (probably a version of blind man's bluff), where he is tricked by his friends, he is deceiving himself in love. He resolves in future to cease this self-deception but, alas:

> [...] soubdain ie m'en accuse,
> Et, maulgré moy, il me faut cheuecher.
>
> [[...] suddenly I find myself guilty of it
> And, despite myself, I must owl (?)].
>
> D57, 9–10

Saulnier suggests that *chevecher* must refer here to the hoot of an owl ("une cheveche"). He supplies a passage from Pedro Mexía (translated by Claude Gruget) to the effect that if owls sing while it is raining, it presages sunshine; when they do so during sunshine, it foretells rain. Thus the poet always tends towards the opposite of his current situation.[37] McFarlane disagrees, proposing that the verb more plausibly derives from another meaning of "cheveche"—a piece of headgear of the kind possibly used to blindfold the players in a game of "Mousche" (1.1): Scève, far from removing the blindfold of his self-deception, is condemned repeatedly to wear it. Montferran's recent study decides in favour of Saulnier's reading, noting the proximity of *chevecher* (D57) to *(se) paonner* (D58) in the subsequent *dizain*: the two cases form a narrative micro-sequence, which may also include another nearby ornithological reference—the "Aigle" of D55, a veiled reference to the imperial ambitions of the Emperor Charles V, eventually transformed into an "Austruche errante." The Saulnier-Montferran reading seems the likelier overall; none the less, *chevecher* remains difficult to pin down exactly. Even if the reader decides that the parent concept is OWL, the precise force of the comparison has still to be determined: Saulnier's thesis has its merits, but *chevecher* could just as plausibly mean "to hoot plaintively" or even "to live a sleepless, nocturnal existence." Gérard Defaux, citing a letter from Guillaume Briçonnet to Marguerite de Navarre, additionally suggests that the owl may refer at once to the (diurnal) blindness of the lover, not forgetting that the owl is an emblem of Minerva: "Ce que donc nous montre ici la *cheveche*," he concludes, "c'est le paradoxe de l'aveugle qui voit, et du voyant qui est aveugle."[38] The sheer range of possible readings, or "weak implicatures," made available by *chevecher* is a telling consequence of underspecification in denominal verbs.[39]

Let us return to Dizain 1 where, although the parent noun of "girouettoit" is not in doubt, the operation of the weather-vane as described elsewhere in *Délie* may not sharpen but actually complicate the movement of *girouetter*:

> L'Œil trop ardent en mes ieunes erreurs
> Girouettoit, mal cault, à l'impourueue:
>
> D1, 1–2
>
> [The too ardent eye of my youthful errors weather-vaned, heedless and at random.]

As mentioned above, this denominal finds a visual analogue in Emblem XV, "La Girouette." But there is a difference: in the emblem the most salient feature of the "girouette" is its *im*mobility. The motto reads "Mille revoltes ne m'ont encore bougé": the image thus serves as a metaphor for the poet's faithfulness in love, with the poet compared in this case not to moving parts but the rigid stem, standing firm despite the winds of fortune or temptation. The poet returns to this stasis-in-motion in the explanatory *dizain* immediately following the image, which ends:

> Parquoy souuent en maintz lieux il [Amour] me trœuve
> Ou audeuant me presente vn obiect
> Avec si doulx, & attrayant subiect,
> Que ma pensée, a peu pres s'y transmue,
> Bien que ma foy, sans suyure mon proiect,
> Cà, & là tourne, & point ne se remue.
>
> D132

> [And so often where love presents before me an object with good reason for appearing kind and attractive, that my thought is almost transferred to it, even though my faith, which does not follow my thought, turns this way and that, and does not move.]

By contrast in Dizain 1 the qualifying adverbs "mal cault" and "à l'impourueu" suggest that the poet's eye has more in common with the fickle revolving blade than the fixed point at the centre. He is recalling his wayward desires before Délie fixed his gaze on her, and only her. Here we need to acknowledge Ellen Spolsky's claim that kinesic understanding may sometimes "compete, rather than cooperate, with other structures of information."[40] Although the final product is reasonably clear, the cognitive work required elicits—here at the very threshold of the sequence—the level of alertness, and kinesic attunement, the reader will require as she enters the weird imaginary ecology of the *Délie* as a whole.

The concluding part of this essay assesses Sébillet's remark on the dynamizing effect—the *energia*—of Scève's neologisms across a whole poem. Take the case of Dizain 99:

> Fusse le moins de ma calamité.
> Souffrir, et vivre en certaine doubtance:
> J'aurois au moins, soit en vain, limité.
> Le bout sans fin de ma vaine esperance.
> Mais tous les jours gruer soubz l'asseurance,
> Que. ceste fiebvre aura sa guerison,
> Je dy, qu'espoir est. la grand prurison,
> Qui nous chatouille à toute chose extreme,

> Et qui noz ans use en doulce prison,
> Comme un Printemps soubz la maigre Caresme.
>
> [Were the least part of my misfortune to suffer, and live in certain doubt: I would at least, though vainly, have brought short the end without end of my vain hope. But every day to crane under the certainty that this fever will have its cure ... I say that hope is the great itch, tickling us in every extreme thing, and which consumes our years in a sweet prison, like a Spring under meagre Lent.]

"Une grue" is a crane, a slightly undignified bird close in appearance to a heron or a stork and which, like these other birds, often spends its time immobile, balanced on one leg. The harsh-sounding *gruer* is another of Scève's neologisms. Saulnier considers a range of possible meanings: "faire l'imbécile," citing Henri Estienne ("Nous usons de ce mot de *grue* en ceste mesme signification de *sot*. Car *c'est une grue* vaut autant que *c'est un sot*"); "faire l'intelligent" (the crane appears in Erasmus and Maurice de La Porte as byword for prudence or careful consideration); or "chasser la grue" ("go crane-hunting"—an exceptionally difficult pursuit to judge by an emblem of Alciatus). Eventually Saulnier resolves that by analogy with the modern French phrase "faire le pied de grue" (already attested in 1544, though only just), we are probably to infer a certain mode of being in one's body: one in which that body waits, fruitlessly, for hours on end.[41] The preposition helps: "*soubz* l'asseurance" (my emphasis) suggests that the poet's attitude has been imposed, as it were from above, by his misplaced certainty: he is sure that, if he waits long enough, he will be cured of his pain. Here again Scève's language prompts a kinesic attunement to bodily posture, to the distribution of weight across space, and perhaps also to corporeal discomfort. But the degree to which this prompt arrives immediately or pre-reflectively is questionable, to say the least. Like many of the verbs discussed by Clark and Clark, the relation of *gruer* to its parent noun remains obscure. The fact seems underlined by the English denominal *to crane*. As with the divergent pairing *to monkey* and *singer* mentioned above, the two languages imagine the same parent noun quite differently: whereas French *gruer* calls our attention to the bird's elongated legs, English *crane* picks out a quite different part of its anatomy (*crane one's neck*).

Structurally speaking, Scève has made "gruer" the fulcrum of his poem. Line 5 is the pivot of a *dizain* with the common 4+6 division, operating something like the *volta* in a sonnet: Scève's denominal occupies its exact syllabic centre. Around this hinge turns the argument of the poem: that the dull constancy of doubt is preferable to itchy, ticklish hope. Itself part-verb, part-noun, "gruer" effects this transition by bridging between the static infinitives of the first half ("souffrir" and "vivre") and the more dynamic nominal sequence with which the poem ends. "Gruer" generates an extraordinary sequence of phonetic and graphic modulations, morphing first into "guerison," then (via "grand") "prurison," "prison," and "Printemps," before the original consonantal cluster returns (twice) with the last words, "maigre Caresme." There seems something very deliberate about this series, which recalls the wordplay of the earlier Grand Rhétoriqueurs, as occasionally happens in Scève. But to insist only on this, or find in it simply another instance of the graphic unconscious or play of the signifier, would be to downplay the effect of "gruer" as a *cognitive* event. In keeping with an aesthetic principle common to many Renaissance artworks, Scève's coinage builds this poem from the centre out.

The echoic energy just mentioned find an analogue in the kinesic force of Scève's denominal verb. Even at the first attempt, most readers will access fairly easily the metaphorical sense of fruitless waiting, possibly via "faire le pied de grue." Compared to that more fully explicated phrase, however, *gruer* requires an increased degree of inferential effort, with the result that the literal component—the crane—arguably lingers at a far higher level of kinesic activation.[42] The afterimage of the poet-crane is strikingly hard to shake off, and continues to induce a kinesic response long after the metaphorical sense—to wait fruitlessly—has faded. Thus in some measure it continues to be this creature, alongside the generalized "nous," whom some readers may imagine as prey to the "prurison" of lines 6–7: "Je dy, qu'espoir est la grand prurison,/Qui nous chatouille à toute chose extrême." Hope is afflicting the poet's skin, hot under his feathers.

The contrast between this hyperaesthesia and the crane's congenital stillness becomes an image of sexual frustration far more specific than the vaguely Petrarchan "doulce prison" (l.9) suggests on its own. The kinesis it induces is similar to—but interestingly distinct from—that of the urticarial itching evoked another of Scève's *dizains*, the more famous D161. There the poet describes himself as wallowing in nettles ("Couvert d'ennuy je me veaultre en l'Ortie"): "se veaultrer" (to wallow) suggests self-indulgence, assent to one's torment; in contrast the upright, rigid crane strives to keep his dignity, even if he fails.[43] Some might want to take this reading further. The noun "grue" has another meaning—"prostitute":

this sense was probably backformed from the posture of one-legged loitering. Were readers to access this meaning first, "chatouille" and "prurison" might begin to suggest the skin conditions brought on by venereal disease. In its phonetic structure, its kinesic richness and in the polyvalency of its nominal stem, "gruer" detonates a poem as vivid as it is unamenable to paraphrase.

Conclusion

Denominal verbs provide the basis for an exchange in the well-known cartoon strip Calvin and Hobbes:

CALVIN:	I like to verb words.
HOBBES:	What?
CALVIN:	I take nouns and adjectives and use them as verbs ... Remember when 'access' was a thing? Now it's something you *do*. It got verbed.
CALVIN:	Verbing weirds language.
HOBBES:	Maybe we can eventually make language a complete impediment to understanding.[44]

Calvin and Hobbes might here be thought to take up positions similar to the ones of Thomas Sébillet and Étienne Pasquier described at the outset of this essay. Calvin (Sébillet) recognizes—and seems to enjoy—the capacity of "verbing" to confer a mysterious energy on language. Meanwhile Hobbes (Pasquier) suggests that "weirding" belongs at one end of a slope that may eventually fall off into exasperating obscurity. Rather than take these viewpoints as straightforwardly antithetical, though, it seems more plausible to suppose that each individual instance will belong somewhere on a gradient between them. We might agree with Calvin that "verbing weirds" the language of the *Délie*, but without conceding to Hobbes that this necessarily results in an "impediment to understanding." Scève's denominal verbs line up on a continuum extending between cases in which we reach the correct inference automatically and ones requiring the far more deliberative operation of kinesic (and not only kinesic) intelligence. At the more straightforward end, this essay has considered *se paonner*; *sagetter* (D268) or *déluger* (D50) would be other examples. Further up the weirdness gradient we find *girouetter* and, occurring shortly after the "Girouette" emblem (XV), we might have mentioned its close cousin *pyrouetter* (from "pyrouet"—a spinning top; D137). Scève invests this verb with added peculiarity by using it transitively, in a description of l'Aveugle (i.e. Cupid) "pyrouettant sur moy ses falleboudes." *Chevecher* is probably the most vexed instance, with *gruer* and perhaps *satyriser* (D104) not far behind. In the end, the range of readings such cases produce—between the reflective and the pre-reflective—underlines the justice of Sébillet's view: of a strange *energia* surfacing unevenly across Scève's "mos nouveaus," and not always most powerful where we grasp their meaning quickest.

Notes

1. "[…] par si estranges façons de parler vous taschez d'obscurcir et ensevelir dans vos vers voz conceptions tellement, que les simples et les vulgaires […] n'y peuvent recognoistre leur langue?"; Pontus de Tyard, *Solitaire premier*, ed. Silvio Baridon (Geneva: Droz, 1950), 67.
2. Ronsard includes Tyard in lists of his notable poetic contemporaries from the 1553 "Élégie à Jean de La Péruse" onwards: he can be found on board ship to the "Isles Fortunées," the New World destination Ronsard imagined for himself and his poet companions in his poem of that title; Pierre de Ronsard, *Œuvres complètes*, ed. Paul Laumonier (Paris: Didier, 1924–1975), 5:180, 261. On Tyard's intellectual relationship to his contemporaries in the early 1550s see especially Eva Kushner, "Le 'Solitaire premier' de Pontus de Tyard: prolégomènes à une interprétation," *Revue belge de philologie et d'histoire*, 50, no. 3 (1972): 760–7.
3. Tyard, *Solitaire premier*, 67–68. All translations from French are my own.
4. On Scève's reputation as a difficult poet, see especially Pascal Quignard, *La Parole de la Délie* (Paris: Mercure de France, 1974); Jerry C. Nash, *The Love Aesthetics of Maurice Scève: Poetry and Struggle* (Cambridge: Cambridge University Press, 1991): ch. 1; François Rigolot, "'Cinq paroles intelligibles': à propos de Scève l'Obscur,'" in *A Scève Celebration:* Délie *1544–1994*, ed. Jerry C. Nash (Saratoga: ANMA, 1994): 55–70.
5. The term "underspecification" has been preferred to "underdetermination" in this essay, in case the latter is confused with (very different) poststructuralist notions concerning the supposed "indeterminacy" of linguistic signs.
6. On "vital signs," see Raphael Lyne's contribution in this volume.
7. On Scève's neologisms, see Henri Weber, *Le Langage de Maurice Scève dans la Délie* (Florence: Publications de l'Institut français, 1948), 8–29; Verdun-Louis Saulnier, *Maurice Scève, italianisant, humaniste et poète (ca. 1500–1560)*, (Paris: Klincksieck, 1948–1949) 1:295–6, 303–4. The most important recent treatment is Jean-Charles Monferran, "Le dictionnaire tout à part soi de

Scève: réflexion sur les mots nouveaux de *Délie*," *Fabula/Les Colloques, Délie, Object de plus haulte vertu* (January, 2013). Accessed 20 December 2016, http://www.fabula.org/colloques/document1803.php

8. The role of the Pléiade in promoting neologism should not be exaggerated. See Halina Lewicka's classic study on neologism and derivation in late-medieval French theatre, *La Langue et le style du théâtre comique français des XVe et XVIe siècles: la dérivation* (Paris: Klincksieck, 1960), 1:361–4.
9. Guillaume des Autels, *Replique aux furieuses defences de Louis Meigret* (Lyon: Jean de Tournes, 1551), 379.
10. Thomas Sébillet, *Art poetique françois* (Paris: Gilles Corrozet, 1548), fol. 9[v].
11. "[...] remains difficult to extract from them [i.e. from his new words]." Sébillet, *Art poetique*, fol. 9[v].
12. Étienne Pasquier, *Les Recherches de la France* (Paris: Laurent Sonnius, 1621), 615.
13. The phrase "co-operative principle" was popularized in 1967 by the philosopher Paul Grice in his influential William James lectures; see Herbert Paul Grice, *Studies in the Way of Words* (Cambridge MA: Harvard University Press, 1989).
14. Richard A. Lanham classes *anthimeria* as a sub-category of *enallage*, and defines it as "using one part of speech for another." He offers the examples "His complexion is perfect gallows" (*The Tempest* 1.1) and "Lord Angelo dukes it well" (*Measure for Measure* 3.2); *A Handlist of Rhetorical Terms*, 2nd ed. (Berkeley: University of California Press, 1991), 13. See also the entry for "conversion" in Katie Wales, *A Dictionary of Stylistics*, 2nd ed. (London: Longman, 2001), 84–5.
15. Maurice Scève, *The Délie of Maurice Scève*, ed. Ian D. McFarlane (Cambridge: Cambridge University Press, 1966). All subsequent references are to this edition, with *dizain* numbers marked in the form D80 etc.
16. Joachim Du Bellay, *Les Regrets; Les Antiquités de Rome*, ed. S. de Sacy (Paris: Gallimard, 1967), 251.
17. On Scève's substantivized infinitives, see especially Gisèle Matthieu-Castellani, "Entre cri et silence: Scève syntaxier," in "Lire Maurice Scève," ed. Françoise Charpentier and Simone Perrier, special issue, *Cahiers textuels* 33/44: 15–25; eadem, "Scève: L'infinitif, la loi, le devenir," in *A Scève Celebration:* Délie *1544–1994*, ed. Jerry C. Nash (Saratoga: ANMA, 1994), 149–60.
18. In other words, English can form denominals using what linguists call "zero affixation/derivation." For an excellent recent study of denominal verb formation across several languages, see Andrew McIntyre, "Denominal Verbs: An Overview," in *Word-Formation: An International Handbook of the Languages of Europe*, ed. Peter Müller, Ingeborg Ohnheiser, Susan Olsen and Franz Rainer (Berlin: De Gruyter Mouton, 2016), 2:1406–23.

On denominal verbs in French, see Christophe Bogacki, "Les verbes à argument incorporé en français," *Langages* 23, no. 89 (1988): 7–26.

19. This view is expressed, for example, in David Crystal, *The Stories of English* (New York: The Overlook Press, 2004), 332. Stephen Pinker claims similarly that "functional shift is one of the processes that make English English."; *The Language Instinct* (New York: Harper Collins, 1994), 181.
20. Louis Guilbert, *La Créativité lexicale* (Paris: Larousse, 1975).
21. Du Bellay, 246.
22. Ronsard, 13:34.
23. Jacques Peletier du Mans, *L'Art poëtique* (Lyon: Jean de Tournes and Guillaume Gazeau, 1555), 39.
24. Henri Estienne, *De la precellence du langage françois* (Paris: Mamert Patisson, 1579), 149–50.
25. Eve V. Clark and Herbert H. Clark, "When Nouns Surface as Verbs," *Language* 55, no.4 (December, 1979): 767.
26. Clark and Clark, 767.
27. Clark and Clark, 768.
28. Bogacki, 7.
29. Clark and Clark, 781.
30. This essay adopts the standard practice in linguistics of capitalizing mental concepts.
31. James J. Gibson, *The Ecological Approach to Visual Perception* (Boston: Houghton Mifflin, 1979), ch. 8 ("The Theory of Affordances").
32. Speakers' tacit knowledge of this range of possibilities is what John Searle calls "the Background." See John Searle, *Intentionality: An Essay in the Philosophy of Mind* (New York: Cambridge University Press, 1983).
33. On expressions such as "to do a Napoleon," which operate similarly to denominal verbs, see especially Herbert H. Clark and Richard J. Gerrig, "Understanding Old Words with New Meanings," *Journal of Verbal Learning and Verbal Behavior* 22 (1983): 591–608.
34. See Marie Lippeveld and Yuriko Oshima-Takane, "Nouns to Verbs and Verbs to Nouns: when do children acquire class extension rules for deverbal nouns and denominal verbs?", *Applied Psycholinguistics* 36, no.3 (2015): 559–588.
35. Deirdre Wilson and Robyn Carston, "A Unitary Approach to Lexical Pragmatics: Relevance, Inference and Ad Hoc Concepts," in *Pragmatics*, ed. Noel Burton-Roberts (London: Palgrave, 2007), 230–59 (237). Relevance Theory goes further than Clark and Clark and considers underspecification an essential feature of almost all linguistic utterances, not just denominal verbs. For a further discussion see Deirdre Wilson, "Relevance and Lexical Pragmatics," *Italian Journal of Linguistics/Rivista di Linguistica* 15, no. 2 (2003): 273–291. I am grateful to Deirdre Wilson for alerting me to these studies.

36. Aside from those already cited, it could be argued that the following emblems all prompt a powerful kinesic response: "L'Homme et le Bœuf" (IV), "Dido qui se brusle" (XIII), "Le Cerf" (XVIII), "Le Bateau a rames froissées" (XXII), "La Selle, & les deux hommes" (XXV), "Le Forbisseur" (XXVIII), "La Cye" (XXIX), "Le Muletier" (XXXII), "L'Asne au Molin" (XXXV), "Europa sur le bœuf" (XXXVIII), "L'Arbalestier" (XXXIX), "Le Mort ressuscitant" (XLIV), "La Femme qui bat le beurre" (XLVII), "Le Chamoys & les chiens" (XLIX).
37. Verdun-Louis Saulnier, "Quelque termes de la langue de Maurice Scève," in *Festgabe Ernst Gamillscheg* (Tübingen: Niemeyer, 1952), 77–91 (78–9).
38. "What the *cheveche* shows us here is the paradox of the blind man who sees, and the seer who is blind." Maurice Scève, *Délie, Objecte de plus haulte vertu*, ed. Gérard Defaux (Geneva: Droz, 2004), 2:88–9. See also Xavier Bonnier, *"Mes silentes clameurs": Métaphore et discours amoureux dans* Délie *de Maurice Scève* (Paris: Champion, 2011), 60.
39. On the relevance-theoretic notion of "weak implicatures," see Billy Clark, *Relevance Theory* (Cambridge: Cambridge University Press, 2013), 235–8.
40. Ellen Spolsky, "Elaborated Knowledge: Reading Kinesis in Pictures," *Poetics Today* 17, no. 2 (Summer, 1996): 162.
41. Saulnier, "Quelque termes," 82–4.
42. For a cognitively inflected treatment of this phenomenon in another difficult poet, see my "The Lingering of the Literal in Some Poems of Emily Dickinson," in *Beyond the Code Model: Reading Literature with Relevance Theory*, ed. Terence Cave and Deirdre Wilson (Oxford: Oxford University Press, forthcoming).
43. This contrast between rigidity (or tension) and relaxation is also a key feature of the passage of Montaigne's "De l'institution des enfans" ("Of the education of children"), discussed by Terence Cave in this volume.
44. Bill Watterson, "Calvin and Hobbes," 25 May 1993.

Bibliography

Bogacki, Christophe. Les verbes à argument incorporé en français. *Languages* 23, no. 89 (1988): 7–26.

Bonnier, Xavier. *"Mes silentes clameurs": Métaphore et discours amoureux dans* Délie *de Maurice Scève*. Paris: Champion, 2011.

Clark, Billy. *Relevance Theory*. Cambridge: Cambridge University Press, 2013.

Clark, Eve C., and Herbert H. Clark. When Nouns Surface as Verbs. *Language* 55, no. 4 (December, 1979): 767–811.

Clark, Herbert H., and Richard J. Gerrig. Understanding Old Words with New Meanings. *Journal of Verbal Learning and Verbal Behavior* 22 (1983): 591–608.

Crystal, David. *The Stories of English*. New York: The Overlook Press, 2004.
Des Autelz, Guillaume. *Replique aux furieuses defences de Louis Meigret*. Lyon: Jean de Tournes, 1551.
Du Bellay, Joachim. *Les Regrets; Les Antiquités de Rome*, edited by S. de Sacy. Paris: Gallimard, 1967.
Estienne, Henri. *De la precellence du langage françois*. Paris: Mamert Patisson, 1579.
Gibson, James J. *The Ecological Approach to Visual Perception*. Boston: Houghton Mifflin, 1979.
Grice, Herbert Paul. *Studies in the Ways of Words*. Cambridge, MA: Harvard University Press, 1989.
Guilbert, Louis. *La Créativité lexicale*. Paris: Larousse, 1975.
Kushner, Eva. Le 'Solitaire premier' de Pontus de Tyard: prolégomènes à une Interprétation. *Revue belge de philologie et d'histoire* 50, no. 3 (1972): 760–67.
Lanham, Richard A. *A Handlist of Rhetorical Terms*, 2nd ed. Berkeley: University of California Press, 1991.
Lewicka, Halina. *La Langue et le style du théâtre comique français des XVe et XVIe siècles: la dérivation*. Paris: Klincksieck, 1960.
Lippeveld, Marie, and Yuriko Oshima-Takane. Nouns to Verbs and Verbs to Nouns: When Do Children Acquire Class Extension Rules for Deverbal Nouns and Denominal Verbs? *Applied Psycholinguistics* 36, no. 3 (2015): 559–88.
Matthieu-Castellani, Gisèle. Entre cri et silence: Scève syntaxier. In *Lire Maurice Scève*, edited by Françoise Charpentier and Simone Perrier. Special Issue, *Cahiers textuels* 33/44 (1987): 15–25.
———. Scève: L'infinitif, la loi, le devenir. In *A Scève Celebration:* Délie *1544–1994*, edited by Jerry C. Nash, 149–60. Saratoga: ANMA, 1994.
McIntyre, Andrew. Denominal Verbs: An Overview. In *Word-Formation: An International Handbook of the Languages of Europe*, edited by Peter Müller, Ingeborg Ohnheiser, Susan Olsen and Franz Rainer, vol. 2, 1406–23. Berlin: De Gruyter Mouton, 2016.
Monferran, Jean-Charles. Le dictionnaire tout à part soi de Scève: réflexion sur les mots nouveaux de *Délie*. *Fabula/Les Colloques, Délie, Object de plus haulte vertu* (February 2013), accessed 20 December 2016. http://www.fabula.org/colloques/document1803.php
Nash, Jerry C. *The Love Aesthetics of Maurice Scève: Poetry and Struggle*. Cambridge: Cambridge University Press, 1991.
Pasquier, Étienne. *Les Recherches de la France*. Paris: Laurent Sonnius, 1621.
Peletier Du Mans, Jacques. *L'Art poëtique*. Lyon: Jean de Tournes and Guillaume Gazeau, 1555.
Pinker, Stephen. *The Language Instinct*. New York: Harper Collins, 1994.
Quignard, Pascal. *La Parole de la Délie*. Paris: Mercure de France, 1974.
Rigolot, François. 'Cinq paroles intelligibles': à propos de Scève l'Obscur. In *A Scève Celebration:* Délie *1544–1994*, edited by Jerry C. Nash, 55–70. Saratoga: ANMA, 1994.

Ronsard, Pierre de. *Œuvres complètes*, edited by Paul Laumonier, 20 vols. Paris: Didier, 1924–1975.

Saulnier, Verdun-Louis. *Maurice Scève, italianisant, humaniste et poète (ca. 1500–1560)*, 2 vols. Paris: Klincksieck, 1948–1949.

———. Quelque termes de la langue de Maurice Scève. In *Festgabe Ernst Gamillscheg*, 77–91. Tübingen: Niemeyer, 1952.

Scève, Maurice. *The Délie of Maurice Scève*, edited by Ian D. McFarlane. Cambridge: Cambridge University Press, 1966.

———. *Délie, Objecte de plus haulte vertu*, edited by Gérard Defaux. Geneva: Droz, 2004.

Searle, John. *Intentionality: An Essay in the Philosophy of Mind*. New York: Cambridge University Press, 1983.

Sébillet, Thomas. *Art poetique françois*. Paris: Gilles Corrozet, 1548.

Spolsky, Ellen. Elaborated Knowledge: Reading Kinesis in Pictures. *Poetics Today* 17, no. 2 (Summer, 1996): 157–80.

Tyard, Pontus de. Solitaire premier, edited by Silvio Baridon. Geneva: Droz, 1950.

Wales, Katie. *A Dictionary of Stylistics*, 2nd ed. London: Longman, 2001.

Weber, Henri. *Le Langage de Maurice Scève dans la Délie*. Florence: Publications de l'Institut français, 1948.

Wilson, Deirdre. Relevance and Lexical Pragmatics. *Italian Journal of Linguistics/ Rivista di Linguistica* 15, no. 2 (2003): 273–91.

Wilson, Deirdre, and Robyn Carston. A Unitary Approach to Lexical Pragmatics: Relevance, Inference and Ad Hoc Concepts. In *Pragmatics*, edited by Noel Burton-Roberts, 230–59. London: Palgrave, 2007.

CHAPTER 5

Metaphor, Lexicography, and Rabelais's Prologue to *Gargantua*

Kathryn Banks

Introduction

Rabelais's fictions offer an excellent testing ground for this volume's claim that renaissance literature can make heightened calls on our kinesic intelligence, inviting complex responses to the language of movement in ways shaped by the cognitive ecology of the Renaissance. Conversely, a cognitive approach grounded in kinesic intelligence has much to offer our understanding of key concerns in Rabelais scholarship, such as friendship, the

I would like to thank the Leverhulme Trust for the award of a Philip Leverhulme Prize, which is funding the research to which my work for this book belongs. This particular essay has been a long time in the making and has incurred a number of debts. I am deeply grateful to Terence Cave, who invited me to be a Research Lecturer in his project "Thinking with Literature," leading me to present research on "kinesic Rabelais" and the *Gargantua* prologue in Durham in 2012 and Oslo in 2013. I am indebted to Ann Moss and to Marc Schachter, who both commented insightfully on drafts of this essay. Finally, thanks are due to participants at our 2014 Kinesis workshop, especially Guillemette Bolens, Neil Kenny and Raphael Lyne.

K. Banks (✉)
Durham University, Durham, UK

K. Banks, T. Chesters (eds.), *Movement in Renaissance Literature*, Cognitive Studies in Literature and Performance,
https://doi.org/10.1007/978-3-319-69200-5_5

body, the relationship between letter and spirit, and various pronounced stylistic traits.[1] This essay addresses two of these issues. It offers fresh insights into the body and its relationship to knowledge in Rabelais. It also casts new light on a striking aspect of Rabelais's style: his tendency to shift playfully between abstract meanings and embodied ones, often by reviving the embodied meanings of either metaphors or Latin etymons. A key claim in this essay is that style should be understood—in part, at least—in cognitive terms, as an indicator of the modes of cognition which the writer utilizes and invites his readers to utilize. I shall suggest that the implications of the stylistic practice studied here are both cognitive and historical. First, Rabelais shifts between calling on embodied cognition to a greater or a lesser extent, in what I term in this essay a "modality switch." Kinesic intelligence is likely to be heightened and may be brought to the level of conscious reflection. Second, the calls Rabelais's "modality switches" make on kinesic intelligence constitute a literary mode of exploring the humanist interest in language as "seamless web," as well as its cognitive implications.[2] To investigate this, I will bring Rabelais's writing into dialogue with the *Commentarii linguae latinae* [*Commentaries on the Latin Language*] composed by Rabelais's Lyonnais contemporary and friend, Etienne Dolet.[3]

The practice of shifting between abstract and embodied meanings is omnipresent in Rabelais's fictions. Indeed, according to François Moreau, Rabelais switches between the "literal" and the "metaphorical" more than any other renaissance writer.[4] Timothy Hampton has analysed some of these "slippages from metaphorical to literal language" to shed light on how literature constructs nationhood.[5] This essay aims to further our understanding of such moves between the "literal" and "metaphorical"; however, I avoid using these terms (except to report other research in its own terms). For a start, Rabelais renews the embodied content not only of "metaphors" but also of Latin etymons. More importantly, it is critical to my argument that what is most cognitively relevant is the *degree* to which abstract or embodied meaning is prominent, for example, the degree to which a "metaphorical" use is lexicalized or, conversely, novel or "renewed." Yet the dominant theories of "metaphor" detract attention from such questions of *degree* by focusing instead on *status* as metaphorical. Ancient philosophers and rhetoricians such as Aristotle, Cicero and Quintilian—from whom both the modern and renaissance periods derive definitions of "metaphor"—concentrate on clearly demarcating metaphor (*translatio*), conceived as the not-proper or the borrowed, from proper meanings (the *proprius,* often translated as the "literal").[6] Modern conceptual metaphor theory differs sharply from the Aristotelian view in emphasizing the pervasiveness of metaphor in our conceptual thinking, yet it too focuses attention on *status as metaphorical* rather than on the *degree* to which metaphor is novel or lexicalized, or the degree to which embodied or abstract meanings are foregrounded. Therefore, this essay for the most part avoids the terms "metaphor" and the "literal," referring instead to degrees of embodiedness or abstraction.

Shifts between embodied and abstract meanings, while found throughout Rabelais's fictions, play a central role in some episodes, often where cognition is a central theme. This essay will examine just one such well known passage, an extract from the prologue to *Gargantua*:

> Crochetastes vous oncques bouteilles? Caisgne. Reduisez à memoire la contenance qu'aviez. Mais veistes vous onques chien rencontrant quelque os medulare? C'est comme dict Platon. *lib. II. de rep.* la beste du monde plus philosophe. Si veu l'avez: vous avez peu noter de quelle devotion il le guette: de quel soing il le guarde: de quel ferveur il le tient, de quelle prudence il l'entomme: de quelle affection il le brise: et de quelle diligence il le sugce. Qui le induict à ce faire? Quel est l'espoir de son estude? Quel bien pretend il? Rien plus qu'un peu de mouelle. Vray est que ce peu, plus est delicieux que le beaucoup de toutes aultres: pource que la mouelle est aliment elabouré à perfection de nature, comme dict Galen. *III. facu. natural.* et. *XI. de usu. parti.*
>
> À l'exemple d'icelluy vous convient estre saiges pour fleurer, sentir, et estimer ces beaulx livres de haulte gresse, legiers au prochaz: et hardis à la rencontre. Puis par curieuse leçon, et meditation frequente rompre l'os, et sugcer la sustantificque mouelle. C'est-à-dire: ce que j'entends par ces symboles Pythagoricques avecques espoir certain d'estre faictz escors et preux à ladicte lecture. Car en icelle bien aultre goust trouverez, et doctrine plus absconce, laquelle vous revelera de tres haultz sacremens et mysteres horrificques, tant en ce que concerne nostre religion, que aussi l'estat politicq et vie oeconomique.
>
> [Have you ever cracked open any bottles? Dawg! Recall to mind your countenance then. But have you ever seen a dog encountering a marrow-bone? It is (as Plato says in Book 2 of *The Republic*) the most philosophical beast in the world. If you have ever seen one, you were able to notice with what dedication it observes it; with what solicitude it guards it; with what fervour it takes hold of it; with what sagacity it cracks it; with what passion it breaks it open, and with what care it sucks it. What induces it to do so? What does it hope for from its assiduity? What good is it aiming at? Nothing more than a bit of marrow. True it is that that *bit* is more delicious than the *ample* of all the rest, since marrow is a nutriment elaborated to its natural perfection (as Galen says *On the Natural Faculties*, Book 3, and *On the Use of Parts of the Body*, Book 11).

> Following that example it behoves you to be wise in order to sniff and smell out and appreciate these beautiful books of high fat, to be swift in pursuit and bold in the attack, and then, by careful reading and frequent meditation, to crack open the bone and suck out the substantificial marrow—that is to say, what I mean by such Pythagorean symbols—sure in the hope that you will be made witty and wise by that reading; for you will discover therein a very different savour and a more hidden instruction which will reveal to you the highest hidden truths and the most awesome mysteries touching upon our religion as well as upon matters of state and family life].[7]

The *Gargantua* prologue has been extensively analysed, especially in the context of debate in the 1980s between literary critics inspired by poststructuralism and those advocating more traditional approaches. That debate centred on whether we were supposed to infer from the prologue that a "substantificial marrow" of "higher" meaning could be derived from Rabelais's fictions, or whether the promise of such a marrow was illusory since meaning was incessantly deferred by the dazzling play of language. However, the passage that evokes the elusive "substantificial marrow" focuses, as much as on the apparent goal of the marrow, on actions which that end goal inspires. It is preceded by the appeal to readers not to be content with the "literal meaning" ("sens literal") but rather to seek a higher meaning ("à plus hault sens interpreter," 6), and followed by the observation that Homer and Ovid were unaware of the meanings that readers would find in their texts (7); however, the passage itself switches to a strong focus on actions demonstrating to readers how they should approach Rabelais's book. Where poststructuralist literary theoretical approaches lent themselves to debating the finality of meaning, a kinesic methodology offers the possibility of analysing in fresh ways Rabelais's emphasis on action.

Critics have noted that the passage insistently represents reading as a bodily activity, comparable for example to gnawing a bone. In contrast, using an approach informed by kinesic intelligence, I shall focus not on the passage's *representation* of reading as embodied but rather on its probable *effects* on the embodied cognition of its readers. Nonetheless, I shall return later to explore the fact that Rabelais invites the cognitive responses under scrutiny precisely when cognition is also the theme of his discussion.

Novel and "Revitalised" Embodied Meanings

The very first word of this passage, *crochetastes*, appears to have been a neologism. The seventeenth-century English translators of the passage, Sir Thomas Urquhart and Pierre Le Motteux, decided that what Rabelais had in mind was picking a lock then stealing a bottle, whereas the twentieth-century translator Michael Screech plumped for "cracking open a bottle."[8] Another possibility might be opening bottles with one's teeth. Indeed while it is obvious that the neologism is a verb, it is not clear what action the verb describes. Therefore, to work out what *crochetaster* might mean, the reader needs to model different candidate movements prompted by the verbs *crocheter* (to open with a hook, or hang on a hook, or open a lock with a hook), and *taster* (to handle, feel, touch, or grope for or to taste, or take an essay of).[9] In other words, the neologism seems likely to make considerable calls on our kinesic intelligence.

This suggestion is supported by a growing body of research indicating that motor responses—or the degree to which they are activated—are context dependent rather than automatic. Importantly for my interests here, the degree of familiarity or novelty of the action-related language seems to play a crucial role. Experiments carried out by Rutvik H. Desai and colleagues strengthen the view that to understand relatively unfamiliar action-related language we use a relatively detailed simulation, whereas, as conventionalization increases, our reliance on sensorimotor systems is reduced.[10] These findings contribute to a "graded view of conceptual embodiment," according to which conceptual representation consists of multiple levels of abstraction from sensory, motor and affective inputs. The top level contains schematic representations that are highly abstracted from detailed representations in the primary perceptual-motor system; these are sufficient for adequate and rapid processing in highly familiar contexts. By contrast, in novel contexts, or when the task requires deeper processing, sensory-motor-affective systems make a greater contribution.[11] So, by creating neologisms, as Rabelais so often did,[12] it seems likely that (at least where the neologisms involved actions) he increased the impact on his reader's kinesic intelligence.[13] Furthermore, in this case at least, given the range of possibilities offered by the combination of *crocheter* and *taster*, it seems likely that readers' responses will constitute not only pre-conscious simulation but also a series of more deliberate rehearsals of the various options. Thus the first line of the extract appeals particularly strongly to our kinesic intelligence.

Then, after this implicit invitation to model the action(s) evoked by *crochetaster*, Rabelais explicitly instructs us to retrieve a simulation of such an action, or to "bring back to memory" our bodily posture when we carried out the action: "Reduisez à memoire la contenance qu'aviez."[14] Thus Rabelais not only invites us to return to bodily experiences, to utilize our bodily cognition, but he is also quite explicit that that is what he is doing. While embodied cognition comes into play without our conscious volition, the instruction to employ it is likely to heighten its effects, and furthermore may prompt some readers to reflect (as Rabelais does) on the fact that they are employing embodied knowledge.

In addition, a secondary meaning of *contenance*—volume or contents, for example of a bottle of wine—may invite us to run a further simulation, given that Rabelais has just asked his readers about an action involving bottles.[15] There are attested examples from before the sixteenth century of *contenance* meaning "volume" or "contents,"[16] and the Latin *contineo* could have hinted at such a sense. So Rabelais may be playing on the polysemy of *contenance*, inviting us to recall not only the various actions suggested by *crochetastes* but also that of consuming the contents of the bottle. In other words, the polysemy of *contenance* offers a further action to recall and to simulate, rendering still more complex the potential use of our kinesic intelligence here. Moreover, since the bottle apparently represents Rabelais's book, its "contents" are, we might assume, precisely what we are aiming to get at through the tricky action(s) denoted by *crochetaster*: the word *contenance* indicates both the supposed goal of our action and also the action or posture itself. In other words, there is perhaps a suggestion that the bodily posture is in some sense the goal and so, on this level too, there is an emphasis on the importance of bodily cognition.

Having thus made strong appeals to our kinesic intelligence, Rabelais then proceeds to a longer description of a set of actions. He begins by inviting us to remember watching a dog eating a bone, rather as he instructed us to retrieve the simulations involving bottles. This prompt to sensorimotor imagining differs insofar as the reader is invited to recall an action he has perceived rather than one he has enacted, yet research suggests that perceiving an action activates our own motor system, even if the action observed (such as chewing a bone as a dog would) is not identical to any action we have ever carried out.[17] The invitation to remember watching a dog eating a bone is followed by a detailed description of what we might have observed. Rabelais uses a wide range of verbs—cracking and sniffing and breaking and sucking and pursuing and attacking. He also describes how each action is carried out, noting that the dog observes the bone with dedication, guards it with care, takes hold of it with fervour, cracks it with affection, sucks it with diligence: "vous avez peu noter de quelle devotion il le guette: de quel soing il le guarde: de quel ferveur il le tient, de quelle prudence il l'entomme: de quelle affection il le brise: et de quelle diligence il le sugce." Michel Jeanneret has observed that this series of verbs referring to canine actions serves, in burlesque fashion, to represent reading as a bodily and physical activity.[18] But, putting the passage's cognitive theme to one side, what about its cognitive effects on its reader? Does the long description of the dog's actions mean that simulating the dog's actions will be an important component of our cognitive response?

None of the verbs employed in the discussion of the dog enjoy the novelty of *crochetaster*. Furthermore, since the dog turns out to be an "example" for the reader, it is clear that Rabelais was calling on the familiar proverbial knowledge according to which extracting marrow meant seeking knowledge (as well as on more general conventional equivalences between eating and knowing[19]). Experiments suggest that, generally speaking, familiar idioms elicit less sensorimotor response than do novel metaphors, which may in turn be less powerful than literal actions: for example, Desai and colleagues observed a "trend of increasing sensory-motor activation from abstract to idiomatic to metaphoric to literal sentences," noting that "when metaphors are very highly conventionalized, as is the case for idioms, engagement of sensory-motor systems is minimized or very brief."[20] However, arguably Rabelais's description of a dog engaging in the multiple actions entailed by pursuing the marrow means that these actions do not lend themselves to being understood in solely abstracted—rather than bodily—ways. In other words, the context in which Rabelais presents the idiomatic marrow estranges the proverb by putting the emphasis back onto bodily experience. In addition, the regular patterning of the long sentence in which the actions are described (the multiple repetition of "de quel(le) [noun] il le [verb]") means that the sentence itself gathers a kind of momentum, a kind of kinaesthetic energy.[21]

To get a sharper sense of the impact of this focus on action in Rabelais's description, we can contrast it with the commentary on a set of related proverbs composed by Rabelais's near-contemporary Charles de Bovelles and published a few years before *Gargantua*:

Mandere ad usque ossa,
Manger jusques aulx os.
Ossa infringere,
Rompre les os.
Eruere medullam,
Tirer la mouelle des os.

Quadrant haec ad plurima. Cum primis ad discumbentium inhonestatem nihil in mensa residui faci[e]ntium pręter ossa, et escam canum. deinde ad principum tyrannidem erodentium plębem. Postremo ad subtiliorem pastum refectionemve esurientis animi. Animus enim rebus in arduis haud literali contentus sensu, nec satis sibi esse ducens solid[a] duntaxat palpare, et erodere ossium substantiam subtili ingenii acumine, ipsa etiam ossium adyta et interiores cryptas adit. Quinimmo ossa refringens latentioris intelligentiae medullam inde eruit, qua esuriem temperet suam, Et inclyte siti medeatur occulta, et arcana quaeque noscendi.

[To eat to the bones.
To break the bones.
To extract the marrow from the bones.

These things allow of several readings. In the first place they refer to the disgraceful behaviour of people at a meal who leave nothing on the table except bones and food for dogs; then to the tyranny of rulers devouring the people; and finally to the more refined food and refreshment for the hungry mind. For the mind, faced with difficult things, is not content with the literal meaning, and concluding that it is not enough for it just to handle material things, and to gnaw the substance of bones with the sharp edge of the intellect, also enters right into the secret chambers and innermost recesses of the bones. And so breaking open the bones it extracts thence the marrow of the more hidden meaning, by which to satisfy its hunger, and to quench in brilliant fashion its thirst for hidden and secret knowledge.][22]

As Michael Screech noted, Bovelles interprets the proverbs with the sense that Rabelais also gives them.[23] And one might observe that Bovelles and Rabelais exploit the same metaphor and also the same basic underlying metaphor (that identified by George Lakoff and Mark Johnson as IDEAS ARE FOOD).[24] However, Bovelles puts much less emphasis on action or movement than Rabelais does. Instead, he sets up a series of parallels: "marrow" means "hidden intelligence," and "tempering hunger" of the mind equates to "finding hidden things." So any activation of embodied knowledge is slight. The passage instead stimulates more strongly an abstracted form of knowledge that replaces marrow with intelligence and eating with finding hidden things. Bovelles decodes the marrow and the eating, making it easier than Rabelais does to understand "extracting marrow" in ways more abstract than bodily. By contrast, Rabelais's focus on describing the dog's multiple actions renews the embodied content underlying the proverbial wisdom, thereby inviting us to think with our bodies.

Furthermore, of course the very fact that the actions are carried out by a dog means that they are not easily understood in purely abstract terms. In addition, the dog's actions appear to offer a gloss or a new perspective on the actions implied by *crochetaster* and *contenance*, especially since references to the two sets of actions are interlaced thanks to the pre-figuring or priming of the dog in the interjection "caisgne" ("bitch"). This complexity makes any easy abstraction of the dog's actions less likely, I think. Readers might instead run and re-run simulations involving both dogs and bottles, so that each set of actions gives a new sense of how the other set is carried out. In short, to use the terms of Jeffrey R. Binder and Desai outlined earlier,[25] Bovelles' commentary invites us to employ schematic representations abstracted from the sensorimotor system, whereas Rabelais elicits a response in which the sensorimotor plays a greater role. Rabelais's renewal of embodied content constitutes a surprising shift, not only from the less embodied discussion that immediately preceded this section of his prologue, but also from what we might have expected "marrow" to mean in such a context.

While the extract as a whole makes a surprising shift to the embodied, on the micro-level of the text, too, there are striking switches between language that is very clearly embodied and language that is less so. These switches are similarly dependent to a large degree on the renewal of the embodied substratum of particular linguistic items. This practice is particularly pronounced in the statement to the reader that "vous convient estre saiges pour fleurer, sentir, et estimer ces beaulx livres de haulte gresse." Readers should be "wise" ("saiges") in order to "sniff" ("fleurer"): the verb "fleurer" clashes with "saiges," making one revisit "saiges" to give it a broader meaning more like that of *sagax*, the Latin term which, in the sixteenth century, was imagined to be its etymon.[26] As Robert Estienne's 1552 *Dictionarium latinogallicum* explains, *sagax* meant having a good sense of smell, and, by extension, being mentally perspicacious, and was associated in particular with the sharp sense of smell in dogs.[27] Thus the shadow of *sagax* behind *saiges* increases the sense that the reader should be sniffing like a dog, engaging in a thoroughly embodied pursuit of "marrow." As on the level of the extract as a whole, as we progress from "saiges" to "fleurer" switches between the more embodied and the less embodied make motor content surprising.

Next, Rabelais lists verbs progressing from *fleurer* through *sentir* to *estimer*. *Fleurer* meant to "smell" or to "sniff."[28] *Sentir* also meant primarily to "smell" or "scent," as well as "to taste,"[29] however, its Latin etymon, *sentire*, which Nicot's 1606 dictionary uses to translate it, meant not only "to discern by the senses" and "to feel, perceive, observe, notice" but also "to think, deem, judge, opine,"[30] meanings that had occasionally appeared in usage of the French verb.[31] The meanings of *estimer*, on the other hand, like those of its Latin etymon *aestimare*, are intellectual rather than sensory.[32] Since it follows *fleurer*, the meanings of *sentir* which would initially come to the fore are its primary sensory meanings; however, the inclusion of *estimer* retrospectively shifts the likely meaning of *sentir*. In short, as the list progresses, it becomes more and more possible to return to a more abstract mode of cognition, to think less of "sniffing" than of something like "judging." However, this is then undercut again when the "livres de haultes" are followed by a physicalized noun, *gresse*, rather than by the abstract noun such as "truth" that the expression would lead us to expect, so that the reader is surprised to find herself sniffing for delicious fat, before then being invited to be "swift in pursuit and bold in attack," rather like a hunting dog. So, within this one sentence, there are striking shifts between the more or less embodied, thanks especially to the renewal of supposed embodied content in *saiges*.

Such switches between embodied and abstract emphasis are omnipresent and striking in Rabelais's writing, often occurring thanks to the revival of the embodied meanings either of Latin etymons like *sagax* or alternatively of French words ("metaphors") that were usually understood with an abstract meaning more than with their previous bodily one. While some of these shifts occur in passing, others generate long passages or even whole episodes, notably that of the frozen words in the *Quart Livre*. Crucially, this is especially the case in passages that explicitly treat questions of knowledge and knowing, such as the one under consideration here. I have focused on the calls the passage makes on the reader's bodily cognition, yet reading is also the theme of the passage. In other words, the practice of shifting in surprising ways between eliciting more abstract or more embodied cognition occurs precisely in concert with the explicit exploration of cognition. Rabelais himself seems to associate the practice with questions about cognition. So, what is at stake cognitively in this practice? What kind of thinking does it elicit and reflect? To offer an answer to this question, I shall begin by turning to Dolet's *Commentaries on the Latin Language*, because, as we shall see, they too foreground moves between the more or less embodied.

Etienne Dolet's *Commentaries* and the Humanist "Language Turn"

Each of Dolet's dictionary entries progresses from the "proper" signification of a word to derived ones, from *proprietas* to *translatio*, or *significatio propria* to *significatio translata*, to use Dolet's terms. This reflects Dolet's interest in derived senses: he asserts that the quality of any language lies less in the proper meanings of its words (*proprietas vocum*) than in the "transferral" of words to other uses or meanings (*translatae dictiones*; *translatio vocum*).[33] In some cases, following the practice outlined in the introduction to his first volume, Dolet gives the *significatio propria* (proper meaning), then the *significatio translata* ("transferred" or derived meaning), then examples of the words used with their proper meaning, then examples of the words used with their derived meaning.[34] Sometimes further distinctions are made so that citations are listed under "proprietatis exempla" ("examples of the proper meaning"), then "translata exempla" (examples of "transferred" or derived meanings), then, for instance, "minus translata exempla" (examples of less "transferred" meanings) and "paulo magis translata exempla" (examples of somewhat more "transferred" meanings).[35] In other entries, Dolet omits such headings, and omits any definitions of derived senses, instead pointing to them only through the quotations listed as examples. Either way, Dolet progresses, more or less gradually, and more or less explicitly, from the proper to the derived. Crucially for my interests here, because of the typical etymological development of Indo-European languages, this often means progressing from the more bodily to the more abstract.[36]

Indeed, while I suggested in my Introduction that the period term *metaphor* (or *translatio*) fails to capture Rabelais's practice, the related period term *translatus* is a closer fit insofar as it is used by Dolet to express an interest in the *more* or *less* derived or *translatus*. Whereas, for Quintilian, there were several kinds of *proprietas*, one of which was opposed to "metaphor" and another to derived meanings,[37] Dolet does not distinguish between metaphor and derived meanings, but rather classifies all meanings that are not *proprius* as *translatus*, and suggests that this status as *translatus* is a matter of degree. Thus, he points to degrees of distance from "proper" meanings to various derived ones, which often implicitly map onto the more or less embodied or abstract. Thus, like Rabelais in his fiction, Dolet in his dictionary entries shifts between the more or less embodied, and draws attention to how abstracted senses have been derived from embodied ones.

To take an example relevant to Rabelais's sagaciously sniffing dog, let us examine the entry for *odorare*:

> ODORARI:
> vel, Odorare.
> ODORARE, et odorari dicimus, et est ex odore aliquid deprehendere, ut odora canum vis: qui ferarum ingressus olfacientes, eas tandem inveniunt.
> Cic. Ad Att. IIII. Tu velim ut Fabium, si quem habes aditum, odorere, istum convivam tuum degustes, et ad me de istis rebus, et omnibus quotidie scribas.
> Ibidem: Soles enim tu haec festivè odorari.
> Idem ad Att. VI. Tu sagacius odorabere.
> Idem: Tu tamen, si quid potes, odorare.
> Idem: Cupio enim antequam Romam venio, odorari diligentius, quid futurum sit.
> Idem: Haec vero eius erat ars, malitia miranda, quod acutissime tota provincia, quidcunque esset necesse, indagare, et odorari solebat.
> Idem: Quò postea quàm venerunt, mirandum in modum canes venaticos diceres, ita odorabantur, et pervestigabant, ut ubi quicquid esset, aliqua ratione invenirent.
> Idem: Odorare tamen Antonii διάθεσιν. quem quidem ego epularum magis arbitror rationem habere, quàm quicquam mali cogitare.
> Idem de Orat. II. Ut odorer quàm sagacissime possim, quid sentiant, quid existiment, quid expectent.[38]

The entry defines *odorare* as "apprehending something through scent, as do hunting dogs who find wild beasts by smell." It then lists nine quotations from Cicero that use the verb in more derived senses. In all the quotations, *odorare* refers to an activity other than literal sniffing of actual scents, yet the degree to which the embodied is to the fore varies. The first citation perhaps increases the salience of sensory pursuit in the verb *odorare* by using it together with *degustare*, which similarly has an embodied meaning, *to taste*, as well as a more abstract one. Other citations, such as the second, fourth, fifth and eighth, in themselves do little or nothing to remind us of the embodied sense of *odorare*. The sixth citation uses the verb as a synonym for *indagare*, which seems more abstract and so may decrease any salience of the embodied and the canine, although perhaps less than we might expect since Dolet's own dictionary entry for *indagare* just a page earlier began by linking that verb to hunting.[39] Then, in stark contrast to some of the earlier citations, as well as to the following one, the seventh uses *odorare* together with *pervestigare*, which—formed on the basis of *vestigium* (*footprint* or *track*)—similarly has a primary sense relating to hunting dogs. Thus Cicero states that those under discussion "scented out" and "tracked" everything. He then adds "you might have thought they were hounds of the chase," thereby strongly underlining the embodied and canine meanings of the two verbs. The ninth and final citation recalls Rabelais's sagaciously sniffing dog since Cicero claims to "sniff out" as "sagaciously" as possible ("sagacissime") the feelings and opinions of jurors[40]; similarly, *sagacius* is used with *odorare* in the third citation. This use of words related to *sagax*—another word with a sensory meaning as well as a more abstract one—probably makes the embodied meaning of *odorare* rather more salient. In short, because all these citations are placed after the embodied and canine definition of *odorare*, and because they recall that definition to varying degrees (especially in the seventh citation), in Dolet's dictionary the verb is presented within its continuum from embodied to abstract senses.

Ann Moss has observed that this method of following the various shades of meaning of an individual word is part of a broader practice on Dolet's part of tracing semantic continua.[41] As well as moving between the *proprius* and the *translatus* within each individual dictionary entry, Dolet traces semantic continua across the sequence of dictionary entries, which he organizes not alphabetically but rather in groups of cognate terms and terms with similar meanings.[42] For example, *odorari* is found within the following sequence: [...] *quaerere*, *explorare*, *expiscari*, *contari*, *scitari*, *sciscitari*, *indagare*, *investigare*, *odorari* or *odorare*, *olfacere*, *scrutari*, *elicere* [...].[43] The sequence moves between words with primarily embodied meanings and words with primarily abstract ones; and, while Dolet often begins these entries with embodied meanings (for example, ones involving hunting in the series *indagare*, *investigare*, *odorari*), in other cases, such as *scitari*, the meanings given are more abstract.

Moss shows that Dolet's tracing of semantic continua between and within his dictionary entries is part of a broader shift in humanist lexicography: whereas the best known scholastic dictionary (the fifth part of the *Catholicon*, which had no serious rival until the early sixteenth century) was concerned with the semantic boundaries of words, humanist lexicographers (particularly more sophisticated ones, such as Valla, Erasmus and Dolet) followed associations between words, creating an "interlocking web" of words.[44] Moreover, Moss argues convincingly that this new attention to semantic continuities was part of a Latin "language turn," a broader humanist change in the use of language that had profound cognitive implications. Dolet himself, to quote Moss, "does not discuss cognitive process" yet "almost, but perhaps not quite, gives to metaphor a creative potential that reaches beyond language to thought"; other humanists were more explicit about the implications of their "webs" of language for thought.[45]

Rabelais probably met Dolet in autumn 1534, when Dolet moved to Lyon. Certainly, from that date they formed a close friendship.[46] By the middle of 1535, Dolet had completed the first volume of his *Commentary*, was seeking royal permission to publish, and had commenced printing.[47] Rabelais's *Gargantua* was probably published in 1535.[48] So, when Rabelais was about to publish *Gargantua*, Dolet was busy with the final stages of producing his dictionary. It is therefore plausible that when Rabelais was still writing *Gargantua* he may have discussed with Dolet the latter's innovative method for compiling a dictionary and the attitude to language that underlay it. But, whether or not such matters were the explicit topic of conversation between the two friends, it seems likely that the humanist interest in the "seamless web" of language would have made Rabelais conscious of, and interested in, the relationship between proper and derived senses of words, and thus between embodied and abstract ones.

Indeed, as we have seen, Rabelais's fictions—and not least his sagely sniffing dog—demonstrate that he was interested in continuities between the embodied and the abstract. Like Dolet, Rabelais explored these continuities on the level of both the individual word and sequences of related words. Rabelais endows the word *saige* with the embodied-abstract continuum of its supposed etymon *sagax*, and associates it, like *sagax*, with the sensory action of hunting dogs. And his series of verbs, "fleurer, sentir, estimer," moves between the more embodied and the more abstract, not unlike Dolet's sequence of entries that moves from *quaerere* through *expiscari* through *scitari* through *odorare*. Moreover, as I noted above, Rabelais's play with more or less embodied or abstract modes of cognition often coincides with explicit discussion of cognition, as in the passage under consideration in this essay. This suggests that it was prompted by an interest not simply in the humanist web of language but also in its cognitive implications: in other words, Rabelais's surprising shifts between the embodied and the abstract explore their possible effects upon thinking. Thus, like some lexicography, Rabelais's fiction constitutes in part a humanist reflection on the cognitive implications of semantic continua.

Thinking with Fiction: Rabelais's "Modality Switches"

This is not to say that Rabelais's French fiction provided the same cognitive affordances—the same tools for thinking—as Dolet's Latin dictionary.[49] Rabelais's text does something different, because it is French and because it is literature. The crux of the matter is that in Rabelais's text the switches to embodied meanings are more striking. For example, the embodied meaning brought to the fore in "saiges," unlike that in the Latin *sagax*, is surprising, as is the embodiedness of "extracting marrow" by cracking and sniffing and sucking. It seems to me that this element of surprise increases the bodily impact on the reader, the effect on the reader's sensorimotor cognition. What support is there for this? Bolens has suggested that the unpredictability of some sensorimotor configurations in literature is key to the power of literary kinesis.[50] But what about, more specifically, the practice I have described?

It is suggestive that, as Ana Raposo and colleagues have shown, action verbs cause more activation in motor regions of the brain if they are encountered in isolation rather than within literal action sentences.[51] Also, as demonstrated by Nicole Speer and colleagues, when comprehending stories, brain regions involved in processing actions increase in activation at points in the narrative when a new goal-focused action is initiated.[52] In other words, at least on the level of pre-conscious cognition, *shifts towards* kinesic content cause greater sensorimotor activation than *sustained* kinesic content does.

Moreover, Anežka Kuzmičová has recently suggested that new motor content is likely to push embodied cognition into conscious experience. Building on Marie-Laure Ryan's research into fictional immersion, Kuzmičová suggests that the transition from non-movement to movement—which she terms a "sudden modality switch"—is likely to bring motor responses to literary texts over the "threshold of consciousness."[53] Kuzmičová, like Speer, is discussing literal movement—shifts from stasis to motion in descriptive passages. However, given the sensorimotor effects of novel metaphors, I would hypothesize that shifts to the embodied from the level of the abstracted etymon or the so-called "dead metaphor" similarly constitute "sudden modality switches" likely to increase sensorimotor response. One wonders if, given insights from Rabelais or other texts, scientists might wish to design an experiment to see if neuroimaging captures any trace of cognitive response to such shifts from the abstracted etymon or "dead metaphor" to the embodied. In any event, reviving the embodied content of metaphors and etymons as Rabelais does certainly seems to cause more surprise than many switches between literal stasis and movement; therefore readers are especially likely to be aware of a sensorimotor response and perhaps to reflect upon the surprising shift that caused it.

In Rabelais's case, it is particularly likely that at least some of his readers would be aware of the shifting calls on their cognition because the passage under consideration (like others in which "modality switches" occur) is explicitly about cognition: while the "modality switches" from embodied to abstract engage our cognition in shifting ways, at the same time Rabelais explicitly invites us to reflect on what reading involves, even flagging up explicitly that we are to use our memory of bodily actions ("Reduisez à memoire" et cetera). Thus the exploration of cognition is multi-faceted: explicit discussion of cognition interacts with an engaging of our cognition in surprising ways, which may elicit our reflection. In addition, a key role in Rabelais's "modality switches" is played by humour: for example, the apparent incongruity of our more embodied reinterpretation of *saiges* with the topic of pursuing knowledge makes us laugh. This humour may prompt kinesic intelligence of a reflective kind: it is likely to make at least some readers reflect on the source of the humour, and thus perhaps bring embodied cognition to conscious awareness and thought.

Rabelais's readers may also have had their kinesic intelligence differently attuned from ours insofar as they were bilingual in Latin. Not much knowledge of Latin is required to recognize the shadow of *sagax* behind Rabelais's use of *saiges*, and perhaps also the trace of the various Latin verbs meaning sniffing and investigating. Moreover, Renaissance readers were more familiar than we are with not only Latin but also the recourse to etymology in definitions of words, used in not only dictionaries but also a range of other discourses.[54] Indeed it is for this reason that Rabelais himself got so much mileage out of the comic etymologies he included in his fictions. In addition, in this particular case, we are dealing with a semantic continuum—from tasting to knowing—which had long been of interest.

Mary Carruthers has recently highlighted the wealth of links made between taste and knowing in both Graeco-Latin and biblical traditions, including the long-standing trope of meditating upon religious texts as "chewing"; indeed, one twelfth-century writer even elaborated on this so that "reading is within the outer skin, meditation in the fat," an image not unlike Rabelais's readerly chewing to get to the fatty marrow. Such links were not understood only as "metaphorical": they stemmed in part from meditation and liturgical practices, as well as the doctrine of the Eucharist itself. And some medieval writers highlighted the double meanings of terms like *sapere*, both *to taste* and *to know*.[55] Moreover, in the Renaissance, in the vernacular as well as Latin, the tasting–knowing continuum came to the fore in new ways, for example, in imitation theory's commonplace images of reading as digestion. In short, then, sixteenth-century readers were more likely to be aware of and to reflect on the relationships between both French and Latin terms for "eating" and "knowing."

Moreover, humanist approaches to language brought renewed and more sustained attention to the relationship between embodied and abstract senses of not only those Latin terms for tasting and knowing but also Latin words in general. Many readers would have been aware of the typical etymological development of words with embodied and abstract senses to ones with only or primarily the latter. So some of Rabelais's readers might have reflected that the bodily actions they are invited to imagine were present in Latin words, which prompted stronger bodily knowing than their French counterparts (and thus, perhaps, gave to bodily knowing something of the venerable status of Latin). Finally, some readers, more aware than others of humanism's "language turn," might have been particularly likely to reflect on the cognitive implications of the semantic continua with which Rabelais presented them.

Conclusion

I have sought in this essay to cast new light on what Moreau and others have termed Rabelais's shifts between the "metaphorical" and the "literal," or what I have described as "modality switches" between the abstract and the embodied, which often work by renewing the bodily content of linguistic items usually understood in a way more abstract than embodied. I have focused attention on readers' probable cognitive responses to this, suggesting that Rabelais shifts between language prompting sensorimotor response to greater or lesser degrees, and that this is likely to enhance kinesic intelligence and, to varying extents, shift it to a conscious and even reflective level. Understanding the relationship between what happens on a pre-conscious level (as measured by neuroimaging) and conscious experience is an extremely thorny problem; however, literature may be especially good at inviting us to become conscious of a continuum between the pre-reflective and the reflective, and at suggesting some ways in which pre-conscious sensorimotor cognition might be pushed to the level of consciousness and even explicit reflection.

Writers in any time and place might play with lexicalized "metaphors" in a way that enhances sensorimotor response and perhaps pushes it over the threshold to consciousness. However, in the early sixteenth century the common human cognitive toolkit was shaped by Renaissance humanism. I have suggested that Rabelais's striking "modality switches" between embodied and abstract were prompted by an interest in the humanist "web" of language and its cognitive implications. Similarly, his readers may have had their kinesic intelligence differently attuned from ours insofar as they were bilingual in Latin, and all the more so insofar as they were aware of humanism's "language turn." The cognitive responses of Rabelais's readers were probably also sharpened by his humour and his foregrounding of the theme of cognition.

The sagaciously sniffing dog and the humanist web of language are, for me, one entry point into a broader exploration of Rabelaisian kinesis in general as well as embodied-abstract shifts more specifically. To explore the latter further, the frozen words episode in the *Quart Livre* is particularly interesting because, as well as engaging in practices like those described in this essay, it also re-embodies precisely *translatio*, turning "metaphor" back into "movement." Such shifts also shed light on the cognitive impact of many of Rabelais's famous lists. But these are questions I hope to address elsewhere. Similar matters might be investigated in other sixteenth-century writers too, since Rabelais was not the only one to re-embody abstract terms, although he did it in his own distinctive way. For example, Montaigne's writing is, as Richard Scholar puts it, "remarkable for the physicality with which it describes abstract processes, an effect it achieves by restoring, to the metaphors it uses, their literal sense."[56] I hope this essay has demonstrated that it is worth examining such practices through the dual lenses of renaissance history and contemporary science.

Notes

1. A different take on kinesis in Rabelais, in particular on friendship, is provided by Michel Jeanneret, another participant in the "Thinking with Literature" project and the Kinesis workshop. "Quand le sens passe par les sens: Rabelais et l'intelligence des corps," *Poétique* 178 (2015): 157–62. See also Timothy Chesters, "Social Cognition: A Literary Perspective," *Paragraph* 37 (2014): 63–71.
2. The expression "seamless web" is borrowed from Ann Moss, *Renaissance Truth and the Latin Language Turn* (Oxford: Oxford University Press, 2003), 49. The notion of a "web" of language is recurrent in Part I ("Words") of Moss's book.
3. Two vols, Lyon: Sebastian Gryphius, 1536 and 1538.
4. *Les Images dans l'œuvre de Rabelais.* Vol. 3: *Un Aspect de l'Imagination créatrice chez Rabelais: l'emploi des images* (Paris: Société d'Édition d'Enseignement Supérieur, 1982), 143–8.
5. "What is most important here for a more general consideration of how literature constructs nationhood are the curious slippages from metaphorical to literal language." For example "[t]hese metaphors may be dead metaphors, but Rabelais brings them to life again, for they are the terms that generate the narrative [...] Panurge's metaphorical description of the Turks as 'treacherous dogs' is neatly literalized." *Literature and Nation in the Sixteenth Century: Inventing Renaissance France* (Ithaca, NY; London: Cornell University Press, 2001), 25, 51. Cf Neil Kenny's suggestion that the Turkish episode discussed by Hampton brings together lambish leanness and other meanings of *curiosus*, demonstrating interestingly that embodied and abstract meanings may be associated because of not only the etymological or metaphorical derivation of abstract meanings from embodied ones but also the gathering together of disparate items under commonplace headings such as *curiosus*. "Plautus, Panurge, and 'les aventures des gens curieux'," in *(Re)Inventing the Past: Essays in honour of Ann Moss*, ed. Gary Ferguson and Catherine Hampton (Durham: University of Durham, 2003), 51–68. Movement between the figurative and the literal in Rabelais has also featured in my own previous research. "'I speak like John about the Apocalypse': Rabelais, Prophecy and Fiction," *Literature and Theology* 26 (2012): 417–38. "Apocalypse and Literature in the Sixteenth Century: The Case of Rabelais and the Frozen Words," in *Visions of Apocalypse: Representations of the End in French Literature and Culture*, ed. Leona Archer and Alex Stuart (Oxford: Peter Lang, 2013), 83–98.
6. According to Aristotle's seminal definition, "metaphor consists in giving the thing a name that belongs to something else" *Poetics*, 1457b. See also Cicero, *De Oratore*, book III 155–69; Quintilian, *Institutio Oratoria*,

book VIII, ch. 6: 1–18. Furthermore, for Aristotle and the rhetoricians, metaphorical status was determined on the level of the individual word, whereas in Rabelais's writing it is on the level of a broader context—a sentence or sequence of sentences—that the degree of prominence of the embodied content is determined.

7. Rabelais, *Œuvres complètes*, ed. Mireille Huchon (Paris: Gallimard, 1994), 6–7. My translation, based on that of M. A. Screech, *Gargantua and Pantagruel* (London: Penguin, 2006), 207.
8. Screech, transl., *Gargantua and Pantagruel*, 207. Urquhart and Motteux, transl., *Gargantua and Pantagruel*, ed. Terence Cave (London: David Campbell, 1994), 20.
9. For *crocheter*, Randle Cotgrave's 1611 English-French dictionary gives "to open, picke open, with a hooke, &c; also, to hang on a hooke," while Jean Nicot's 1606 *Thresor de la langue française* offers "resignare, Unco aperire" and, for "crocheter une serrure," "Unco seram aperire." For *taster*, Cotgrave offers "to tast; or take an eßay of; also, to handle, feele, touch, or grope for," while for *taster, tastonner*, Nicot gives "attrectare, contrectare" but also translates some set expressions (*taster du vin*, and *taster et gouster petit à petit)* in which *taster* refers to tasting, particularly in the context of wine.
10. "These results support a gradual abstraction process whereby the reliance on sensory-motor systems is reduced as the abstractness of meaning as well as conventionalization is increased, highlighting the context sensitive nature of semantic processing." Rutvik H. Desai et al., "A piece of the action: Modulation of sensory-motor regions by action idioms and metaphors," *NeuroImage* 83 (2013): 862. On simulation more generally, see the Introduction to this volume.
11. Desai et al., 868. For a fuller account of this view, see Jeffrey R. Binder and Rutvik H. Desai, "The neurobiology of semantic memory," *Trends in Cognitive Sciences* 15 (2011): 527–36.
12. Leo Spitzer, *Die Wortbildung also stilistiches Mittel exemplifiziert an Rabelais* (Halle: Max Niemeyer, 1910).
13. On neologism and kinesic intelligence, see also Timothy Chesters in this volume.
14. The French word *contenance* referred, then as now, to the bearing of the body as a whole (rather than primarily to facial expression, as its English cognate does). See, for example, the *Dictionnaire du moyen français,* http://www.atilf.fr/dmf/definition/contenance. Cotgrave's translation of *contenance* (presumably under the influence of English) emphasises the face but also makes clear that the word can mean the bearing or movement of the body: "the countenance, looke, cheere, visage, favor; gesture, posture, behaviour, carriage; presence, or composition of the whole bodie."

15. Thanks are due to Marc Schachter for this observation.
16. http://www.atilf.fr/dmf/definition/contenance
17. See Introduction to this volume, pp. 4–5.
18. *Des Mets et des mots: banquets et propos de table à la Renaissance* (Paris: José Corti, 1987), 119–23.
19. See pp. 96–7 in the later section in this essay, "Thinking with Fiction: Rabelais's 'Modality Switches'."
20. "A piece of the action," 862, 867–8. See also Rutvik H. Desai et al., "The Neural Career of Sensory-motor Metaphors," *Journal of Cognitive Neuroscience* 23 (2011): 2376–86.
21. On syntax and kinesis, see Terence Cave's essay in this volume.
22. Bovelles, Charles de, *Proverbiorum Vulgarium Libri tres* ([Paris]: M.P. Vidouaeo, 1531), vol. II, f. lxxiii[v]. In transcribing Latin quotations I have, where relevant, changed *ā* to *an* or to *am*; *ę* to *ae*; *ĕ* to *em*; *i* to *j*; *ī* to *in*; *j* to *i*; *q* to *que*; *ß* to *ss*; *u* to *v*; *ŭ* to *um*; *&* to *et*. In the case of this quotation I have also corrected *faciuntum* to *facientium*, and *solidam* to *solida*. All translations from Latin are my own.
23. *Rabelais* (London: Duckworth, 1979), 129.
24. *Metaphors We Live By* (Chicago: Chicago University Press, 1980).
25. Binder and Desai, "The neurobiology of semantic memory."
26. "Sage, *Sapiens*. Semble qu'il vienne de Sagax" (Nicot, 1606). The etymon of *sage* is now thought to be *sapidus*. Oscar Bloch and Walther von Wartburg, *Dictionnaire étymologique de la langue française* (Paris: Presses Universitaires de France, 2002), first published 1932, 568.
27. "Sagax, sagacis, Cic. Qui ha grand flairement. Et per translationem, Qui conjecture et prevoit bien les choses advenir, Sage, Prudent, Bien advisé. [...] Sagaces canes. Cic. Qui sentent incontinent la trace de la beste, comme font les chiens qu'on appelle espagnols, et autres appelez pendants." Lewis and Short's modern dictionary also notes that the primary meaning of *sagax*, "of quick perception, whose senses are acute, sagacious," is "chiefly of the acute sense of smelling in dogs." The notion that the reader would actually be *sagax* like the dog, rather than merely *saige*, may possibly also be suggested by the presentation of the dog as an "example" rather than a simile, however Erasmus employed "example" with a broad Aristotelian sense that encompassed similitudes, analogies, and so on. Cf for Quintilian, example was the figure of comparison in which the things compared were most similar, hence example was unlike simile when simile compared animals to people (*Institutio Oratoria*, bk 5, ch. 11.22), and sixteenth-century poetic theorists usually gave *example* a limited sense, attributing to it the function of providing models of conduct or models for writing. John D. Lyons, *Exemplum: The Rhetoric of Example in Early Modern France and Italy* (Princeton, NJ: Princeton University Press, 1989), 6–20.

28. The *Dictionnaire du moyen français* gives A. "Répandre une odeur agréable"; B. "Répandre une odeur désagréable, puer"; C. "Percevoir, sentir une odeur." http://www.atilf.fr/dmf
29. Cotgrave gives "to feele; also, to sent, smell, vent, wind; also, to tast or savor; also, to heere; also, to yeeld a sent, savor, or tast; or to sent, savor, or tast, of; to have a smacke, touch, or spice, of."
30. Lewis and Short.
31. http://www.atilf.fr/dmf
32. Cotgrave gives "to esteeme; think, deeme, trowe, suppose, repute, hold; weigh, consider; judge; prise, value; regard, respect, hold deere, set by, make much account of."
33. I do not render "translatus" or "translatio" using terms such as "figurative" or "metaphor" because—as I will discuss—Dolet considers the *translatus* as a matter of degree. "LOCIS multis (id quod tamen maximè in tertio Tomo nostro demonstrabimus, cùm de phrasi Linguae Latinae scribemus) tum in hoc, tum in primo Tomo nostro à nobis traditum est, linguae cuiusvis et usum, et venustatem non in vocum tantùm proprietate, sed in translatis potissimum dictionibus consistere (id quod, inquam, quanta maxima fieri poterit diligentia, et judicio, tertio Tomo nostro docebimus) dignitatemque praecipuam ex vocum translatione linguas omnes nancisci." ["In many places both in this volume and in my first volume (and most of all I will show this in my third volume, when I write about expressions of the Latin language) I have passed on that the use and charm of any language consists not only in the proper meaning of words but most of all in transferred uses of words (that which, I say, I will show in my third volume with the greatest care which is possible, and judgement) and that all languages acquire their particular value from the 'transferral' of words."] (Lyon: Sebastian Gryphius, 1538), vol. II, col. 883.
34. "COMMENTARIORUM meorum ratio tibi ut liquidius, faciliusque constet, quo in his utar ordine, scire te quidem velim. Principio propositae vocis significationem tum propriam, tum translatam ostendimus. Deinde usus varietatem distinguimus. Postremo exempla cumulamus: sed ea separatim. Nempe ut sua proprietati assignentur: translationi deinceps sua. Quod verò ad usus varietatem pertinet, sic nos quoque exempla secernimus, ut statim post dictionis proprietatem, translationemque (si quam fortè translationem habet) quanta possum diligentia, diligenter ostensam simplicia exempla sine intervallo sequantur." ["So that you may more clearly and easily understand the method in my Commentaries, I want you to know the arrangement that I am using in them. First of all I show the meaning of the word under discussion, both its proper and transferred meaning. Then I distinguish its variety of uses. Last of all I pile up examples, but each of these things separately. So that examples are assigned to

the proper meaning and then to the transferred meaning. But in setting forth the variety of uses, I also divide the examples in such a way that immediately after I have carefully shown with as much care as I am able the proper meaning and the transferred meaning of the word (if it has a transferred meaning), simple examples follow without a pause."] "De Commentariorum ratione, et ordine" (Lyon: Sebastian Gryphius, 1536), vol. I, prefatory material, unpaginated.

35. For example, vol. II, cols. 884–5.
36. Meaning more usually moves from concrete to abstract than the reverse. For a discussion of this in relation to Indo-European perception verbs, see Eve Sweetser, *From Etymology to Pragmatics: metaphorical and cultural aspects of semantic structure* (Cambridge: Cambridge University Press, 1990), 23–48.
37. *Institutio oratoria*, book VIII, ch. 2.
38. Vol. I, col. 171.
39. "INDAGARE est venatorum more inquirere, qui loca, ubi ferae latibula habent, investigant: dicimus autem indago rem, vel, de re" (Vol. I, col. 170).
40. The verbs immediately following *odoror* in this citation—"sentiant [...] existiment"—also mean that it bears an interesting similarity to Rabelais's sequence "fleurer, sentir, estimer," although the latter two verbs are not presented as synonyms or equivalents for *odoror* in the Cicero citation and one would not wish to draw firm conclusions from this (almost certainly coincidental) similarity.
41. *Renaissance Truth*, 27–8.
42. As Dolet puts it in the preface to the first volume ("De Commentariorum ratione, et ordine," unpaginated), "Vocabuli verò primò positi proprietate, translatione, usus, constructionisque varietate et verbis nostris, et Ciceronis exemplis satis multis demonstrata, voces alias significationis cognatione superioribus affines actutum subjungo: rem deinde, quantum licet, perpetuo" ["After I have demonstrated both with my own words and with sufficiently many examples from Cicero the proper meaning and transferred meaning and the diversity of use and of arrangement of the word under discussion, I immediately join other words which are connected by kinship to earlier words then I continue this affair for as long as possible."] Dolet draws attention to this practice relatively often, for example, Vol. II. Prefatory "De Secundi tomi ordine," unpaginated; vol. II, cols. 1034, 1085, 1583. In the epitomes of the *Commentarii* produced by a Basle publisher (1537, 1539, 1540), the word entries in the first volume were rearranged alphabetically, although the original order was reproduced in tabular form after the lexicon proper; the second volume retained the arrangement by subject groups. The number of examples was also reduced.

See Moss, 31–2. Dolet himself was proud of the order of his *Commentarii*, expressing this pride not only on a number of occasions in this work but also in others: see Michel Magnien, "La Philologie selon Dolet," in *La Philologie humaniste et ses représentations dans la théorie et dans la fiction*, ed. Perrine Galand-Hallyn, Fernand Hallyn, and Gilbert Tournoy (Geneva: Droz, 2005), vol. II, 449, n. 30.

43. Vol. I, cols. 168–72.
44. Moss, 28.
45. Moss, 30.
46. The sudden rupture in their friendship did not occur until 1542. Mireille Huchon, "Dolet et Rabelais," in *Étienne Dolet 1509–2009*, ed. Michèle Clément (Geneva: Droz, 2012), 345–59. Richard Copley Christie, *Étienne Dolet, The Martyr of the Renaissance 1508–1546: A Biography* (London: Macmillan and Co., 1899), first published in 1880, 371–86.
47. Copley Christie, 229–40.
48. *Gargantua* may have been published in 1534 but Huchon speculates that it is most likely to have been in the first third of 1535. *Œuvres completes*, 1054–55.
49. On literary affordances, see Terence Cave, *Thinking with Literature: Towards a Cognitive Criticism* (Oxford: Oxford University Press, 2016), 46–62.
50. "Literature is powerful because, more than any other type of discourse, it triggers the activation of unpredicted sensorimotor configurations." *The Style of Gestures: Embodiment and Cognition in Literary Narrative* (Baltimore: The Johns Hopkins University Press, 2012), 17.
51. Ana Raposo et al., "Modulation of motor and premotor cortices by actions, action words and action sentences," *Neuropsychologia* 47 (2009): 388–96.
52. Nicole K. Speer et al., "Reading Stories Activates Neural Representations of Visual and Motor Experiences," *Psychological Science* 20 (2009): 989–99.
53. Kuzmičová, "Presence in the reading of literary narrative: a case for motor enactment," *Semiotica* 189 (2012): 23–48. Ryan, *Narrative as Virtual Reality: Immersion and Interactivity in Literature and Electronic Media* (Baltimore: The Johns Hopkins University Press, 2001).
54. Drawing attention to this, Judith Anderson argues that we should "free Renaissance meaning from narrow, anachronistic lexicalisation." Anderson also observes that Robert Estienne's 1532 *Thesaurus linguae latine* draws attention to the principle of *translatio*. It does so in a less explicit and nuanced way than Dolet's *Commentaries*. "Translating Investments: The Metaphoricity of Language, 2 Henry IV, and Hamlet," *Texas Studies in Literature and Language* 40 (1998): 231, 235; reproduced in *Translating Investments: Metaphor and the Dynamic of Cultural Change in Tudor-Stuart England* (New York: Fordham University Press, 2005), 8–35.

55. Carruthers, *The Experience of Beauty in the Middle Ages* (Oxford: Oxford University Press, 2013), 80–134. "Lectio in cortice, meditatio in adipe" (Guigo II, *Scala claustralium,* 3.43–7; cited by Carruthers, 131, n. 49).
56. *Montaigne and the Art of Free-Thinking* (Oxford: Peter Lang, 2010), 73. See Terence Cave in this volume.

Bibliography

Anderson, Judith. Translating Investments: The Metaphoricity of Language, 2 Henry IV, and Hamlet. *Texas Studies in Literature and Language* 40 (1998): 231–67.

———. *Translating Investments: Metaphor and the Dynamic of Cultural Change in Tudor-Stuart England.* New York: Fordham University Press, 2005.

Banks, Kathryn. Apocalypse and Literature in the Sixteenth Century: The Case of Rabelais and the Frozen Words. In *Visions of Apocalypse: Representations of the End in French Literature and Culture*, edited by Leona Archer and Alex Stuart, 83–98. Oxford: Peter Lang, 2013.

———. 'I Speak Like John about the Apocalypse': Rabelais, Prophecy and Fiction, *Literature and Theology* 26 (2012): 417–38.

Binder, Jeffrey R., and Rutvik H. Desai. The Neurobiology of Semantic Memory. *Trends in Cognitive Sciences* 15 (2011): 527–36.

Bloch, Oscar, and Walther von Wartburg. *Dictionnaire étymologique de la langue française.* Paris: Presses Universitaires de France, 2002.

Bolens, Guillemette. *The Style of Gestures: Embodiment and Cognition in Literary Narrative.* Baltimore: The Johns Hopkins University Press, 2012.

Bovelles, Charles de. *Proverbiorum Vulgarium Libri tres.* Paris: M.P. Vidouaeo, 1531.

Carruthers, Mary. *The Experience of Beauty in the Middle Ages.* Oxford: Oxford University Press, 2013.

Cave, Terence. *Thinking with Literature: Towards a Cognitive Criticism.* Oxford: Oxford University Press, 2016.

Chesters, Timothy. Social Cognition: A Literary Perspective. *Paragraph* 37 (2014): 62–78.

Copley Christie, Richard. *Étienne Dolet, The Martyr of the Renaissance 1508–1546: A Biography.* London: Macmillan and Co., 1899.

Desai, Rutvik H., Lisa L. Conant, Jeffrey R. Binder, Haeil Park, and Mark S. Seidenberg. A Piece of the Action: Modulation of Sensory-Motor Regions by Action Idioms and Metaphors. *NeuroImage* 83 (2013): 862–69.

Desai, Rutvik H., Jeffrey R. Binder, Lisa L. Conant, Quintino R. Mano, and Mark S. Seidenberg. The Neural Career of Sensory-motor Metaphors. *Journal of Cognitive Neuroscience* 23 (2011): 2376–86.

Dolet, Etienne. *Commentarii linguae latinae*. 2 vols. Lyon: Sebastian Gryphius, 1536 and 1538.

Hampton, Timothy. *Literature and Nation in the Sixteenth Century: Inventing Renaissance France*. Ithaca, NY: Cornell University Press, 2001.

Huchon, Mireille. Dolet et Rabelais. In *Étienne Dolet 1509–2009*, edited by Michèle Clément, 345–59. Geneva: Droz, 2012. Cahiers d'Humanisme et Renaissance 98.

Jeanneret, Michel. *Des Mets et des mots: banquets et propos de table à la Renaissance*. José Corti, 1987.

———. Quand le sens passe par les sens: Rabelais et l'intelligence des corps. *Poétique* 178 (2015): 147–62.

Kenny, Neil. Plautus, Panurge, and 'les aventures des gens curieux.' In *(Re)Inventing the Past: Essays in Honour of Ann Moss*, edited by Gary Ferguson and Catherine Hampton, 51–68. Durham: University of Durham, 2003.

Kuzmičová, Anežka. Presence in the Reading of Literary Narrative: A Case for Motor Enactment. *Semiotica* 189 (2012): 23–48.

Lakoff, George, and Mark Johnson. *Metaphors We Live By*. Chicago: Chicago University Press, 1980.

Lyons, John D. *Exemplum: The Rhetoric of Example in Early Modern France and Italy*. Princeton, NJ: Princeton University Press, 1989.

Magnien, Michel. La Philologie selon Dolet. In *La Philologie humaniste et ses représentations dans la théorie et dans la fiction*, edited by Perrine Galand-Hallyn, Fernand Hallyn, Gilbert Tournoy, vol. II, 439–62. Geneva: Droz, 2005.

Moreau, François. *Les Images dans l'œuvre de Rabelais. Vol. 3: Un Aspect de l'Imagination créatrice chez Rabelais: l'emploi des images*. Paris: Société d'Édition d'Enseignement Supérieur, 1982.

Moss, Ann. *Renaissance Truth and the Latin Language Turn*. Oxford: Oxford University Press, 2003.

Rabelais, François. *Œuvres complètes*. Edited by Mireille Huchon. Paris: Gallimard, 1994a.

———. *Gargantua and Pantagruel*. Translated by Sir Thomas Urquhart and Pierre Le Motteux, edited by Terence Cave. London: David Campbell, 1994b.

———. *Gargantua and Pantagruel*. Translated by M. A. Screech. London: Penguin, 2006.

Raposo, Ana, Helen E. Moss, Emmanuel A. Stamatakis, and Lorraine K. Tyler. Modulation of Motor and Premotor Cortices by Actions, Action Words and Action Sentences. *Neuropsychologia* 47 (2009): 388–96.

Ryan, Marie-Laure. *Narrative as Virtual Reality: Immersion and Interactivity in Literature and Electronic Media*. Baltimore: The Johns Hopkins University Press, 2001.

Scholar, Richard. *Montaigne and the Art of Free-Thinking*. Oxford: Peter Lang, 2010.

Screech, Michael A. *Rabelais*. London: Duckworth, 1979.

Speer, Nicole K., Jeremy R. Reynolds, Khena M. Swallow, and Jeffrey M. Zacks. Reading Stories Activates Neural Representations of Visual and Motor Experiences. *Psychological Science* 20 (2009): 989–99.

Spitzer, Leo. *Die Wortbildung also stilistiches Mittel exemplifiziert an Rabelais*. Halle: Max Niemeyer, 1910.

Sweetser, Eve. *From Etymology to Pragmatics: Metaphorical and Cultural Aspects of Semantic Structure*. Cambridge: Cambridge University Press, 1990.

CHAPTER 6

The Gunpowder Revolution in Literature: Early Modern Wounds in Folengo and Rabelais

Guillemette Bolens

This essay begins with a desire to account for two strange wounding gestures in Folengo's and Rabelais's literary works. The attempt to understand these gestures will take us into a discussion of one of the most radical technological changes of the sixteenth century, the so-called Gunpowder Revolution, and the profound changes it prompted in both the nature of warfare and the cultural understanding and representation of the human body in literature. The first of these wounding gestures, in Folengo's *Baldo* (1517/1552), consists in a character using Adam's Edenic apple as a cannonball propelled to kill.[1] The second, in Rabelais's *Gargantua* (1534), involves striking and dismantling enemies by means of the shaft of the Cross. By focusing on such peculiar narrated movements, I wish to emphasize the distinction made in early modern literature between the act of *striking* and the act of *shooting*. Indeed, these two types of action and their related kinesic verbs were invested with moral values at a time when the gunpowder revolution was progressively changing warfare practices, the experience of embodiment and kinesic imagination.[2] In Folengo, the epic hero Baldo fights against an army of devils. His superiority is manifest in

G. Bolens (✉)
University of Geneva, Switzerland

K. Banks, T. Chesters (eds.), *Movement in Renaissance Literature*, Cognitive Studies in Literature and Performance,
https://doi.org/10.1007/978-3-319-69200-5_6

that he never uses artillery, unlike his evil adversaries. He strikes rather than shoots. Meanwhile, the impact of his powerful hand on his enemies' bodies is ultimately that of an explosion. In Rabelais, Frère Jean withstands the attack of the Close of the abbey of Seuilly by Picrochole's ransacking troops in a memorable and detailed act of mass slaughter, performed by means of the shaft of the Cross. In both Folengo and Rabelais, the hero strikes rather than shoots, but his blows end up being as destructive as gunpowder. My purpose is to understand such narrated gestures and highlight their significance in early modern literature.

In "Elaborated Knowledge: Reading Kinesis in Pictures," Ellen Spolsky writes:

> All understanding is a result of interpretation, from identifying object boundaries to reading literary texts, and all interpretation is cognitively continuous. Aesthetic judgments are not different knowledge so much as elaborated inferences produced at one end of a scale of complexity. The quantum advantage to the organism of having a variety of windows on the world, even when those windows produce gaps that must be filled inferentially, is that those gaps are the loci of creativity. Not only is there no need for all systems to be entirely translatable into one another, but such an arrangement would actually be a disadvantage because it would be entirely rigid. It would close all possibility of reaction to new situations, or to old situations in new ways. The gaps in the system—the places where inferences must be constructed—are sites of productive indeterminacy in all brain functions.[3]

The potentials of a productive indeterminacy may be thought to be at work when Folengo and Rabelais react in their art to the disturbing situations elicited by the gunpowder revolution. Through fiction, they invest new meanings in already powerful symbols, such as the Edenic apple and the Christian cross. I will claim that Rabelais in particular does so in order not so much to condone violence as to raise the problem of mass violence, in all its concrete and kinesic implications.[4]

According to J.R. Hale:

> Portable firearms and artillery came radically to affect the conduct and conditions of war. For the soldier they changed the equipment he wore and carried; the formations which affected his morale and practice in combat; the nature of his wounds, for they broke bones and led to loss of limbs by gangrene; and, more conjecturally, his chances of being killed.[5]

Concerning literature, Michael Murrin writes in *History and Warfare in Renaissance Epic* that the gun posed a problem for the writers of romance and epic that had no parallels in tradition. Crossbows and the heavier armour they necessitated or the enceinte castles of the thirteenth century had not much altered the romancers' craft. But writers in the fifteenth and early sixteenth centuries were faced with the new technology of firepower, developed between 1440 and 1530. The use of the gun in warfare challenged the basis of their fictions and provoked strong responses.[6]

Murrin explains how the "Olimpia episode in Ariosto's *Orlando furioso* [1516/1532] presented the negative critique of the gun in its classic form and set the model for writers outside of Italy," later including Milton.[7] Namely, firearms are for cowards, who shoot from a distance instead of meeting their adversaries in close contact and in a spirit of fair play. But, as Murrin notes, distance weapons were hardly new in the sixteenth century: the use of slings, javelins, thrown spears and bows had been a feature of warfare for centuries, and more recently heavy crossbows had given them greater destructive power. What made portable firearms and handguns so troubling was the fact that they placed devastating destructive power into the hands of combatants alien to the chivalric circle of elite heroism, who might bring to the narrative of knightly combat the kinds of destructiveness hitherto associated only with magical or superhuman prowess. The prospect of such enticing yet horrific power in such hands created an ideological dilemma for writers of the early part of the sixteenth century. For example, in the passage of *Baldo* that we will consider, Folengo echoes Ariosto's negative opinions on guns, while his fiction adds a level of complexity to the matter.[8] Indeed, Baldo, being heroic and praiseworthy, does not use firearms, and yet he manages nonetheless to reproduce their catastrophic physical impact. Through a deft manoeuvre, Folengo registers the spectacular impact of the gunpowder revolution in his text without compromising his hero's chivalric identity as a consequence.

In the general context of the long-lasting Great Italian Wars (1494–1559), Folengo and Ariosto were both writing just a few years after the battle of Ravenna in 1512, where France and the Duchy of Ferrara fought against Spain and the Papal States. According to Murrin, "Ravenna was perhaps the bloodiest battle of the century. Fourteen thousand people died."[9] Murrin quotes Jacopo Guicciardini describing it to his brother: "It was a horrible and terrible thing to see how every shot of the artillery made a lane through those men-at-arms [the Spanish heavy cavalry], and how helmets with the heads inside them, scattered limbs, halves of men, a vast quantity, were sent flying through the air."[10] Although Folengo condemns firearms for allowing cowards to murder commendable men from afar, he also describes Baldo's action in ways that resonate with the above description: "[I]t is satisfying to describe some of Baldo's blows ["iuvat alquantos Baldi describere colpos"]. [...] With the point of his blade, he lops off the arms, legs and horned heads of these infernal soldiers and makes them flap through the skies" ["at maxime puntis,/spiccat ab Inferni soldatis brachia, gambas,/cornutasque facit volitare per aëra testas"] (XIX, 319–21). The enemies of Baldo in this passage are devils, but Folengo's hero inflicts his violence on humans with equal gusto and efficacy. The important point is that he uses his sword or his bare hands to achieve such effects, not guns.

More than against artillery in general, Ariosto reacted against the development of the harquebus, "which immediately preceded the composition of the Olimpia episode, [and] gave rise to his moral analysis that modern technology was incompatible with chivalry."[11] Folengo proffers similar arguments. Despite the fact that his work is often parodic, meshing extreme vulgarity with chivalric claims in ways that make any clear-cut moral assessment unwieldy, his objection to the harquebus is unambiguous. Kelly DeVries and Robert Douglas Smith explain that "by the closing decade of the fourteenth and the beginning of the fifteenth centuries a wide range of gunpowder artillery had developed, from small handguns and large battlefield pieces to huge siege guns."[12] While the "hand cannon was a clumsy weapon, and a thoroughly inaccurate one," the harquebus "had much greater possibilities":

> A metal tube, mounted on a wooden stock and fired from the shoulder, by means of a touchhole and a match device, it was not a difficult weapon to handle. Its ball had considerable penetrating power, and it was accurate.[13]

Again, the damage the harquebus was liable to cause did not match nor guarantee the courage and moral merit of its owner. Thus firearms changed the rules of the game.

> The invention of gunpowder weapons had an impact not only on warfare, but on society and the state as well. Most knights, nobles, and princes seem not to have welcomed the introduction of gunpowder weapons. Traditional medieval warfare respected their social status, leading frequently to ransom rather than death following capture. But gunpowder weapons had no such respect for class, and nobles risked death as much from gunshot as did non-noble soldiers.[14]

Fiction evinces reluctance to accept such facts by staging heroes impervious and immune to firearms. In Folengo, cannonballs never actually reach Baldo, and in Rabelais, Gargantua is too gigantic to be harmed by them. Gargantua is shot with cannons, falconets and harquebuses at the Chasteau du Gué du Vede. Once he has had explained to him that the projectiles he feels hitting his head (all shooters are aiming at his head) are neither gadflies nor grape-pips, he takes a massive tree and razes the castle to the ground, crushing those inside to pieces: "Par ce moyen feurent tous rompuz et mis en pieces ceulz qui estoient en icelluy" ["By which means all inside were crushed and smashed into smithereens"].[15] Gargantua's suprahuman physicality achieves the type of destruction expected from bombards and cannons—albeit by striking (with a tree), not shooting—while he himself is impervious to the effect of the enemy artillery.

When Gargantua later combs his hair, making numerous cannonballs fly from his head, his father Grandgousier asks whether these are fleas, which he calls "les éperviers de Montagu" ["the sparrow-hawks of Montaigu]," that is, the fleas plaguing students in the college of Montaigu, ruled by the infamously cruel Beda. Beyond the general humour of the scene, Ponocrates' prompt reaction conveys serious overtones: had he been the king of Paris, he would have burned this college to ashes for the cruelty inflicted on its students, and with it its principal and regent "qui endurent ceste inhumanité davant leurs yeulx estre exercée" (103) ["who tolerate such inhuman behaviour before their very eyes"] (321). The humour of a giant mistaking cannonballs for thrown grapes thus leads to a protest against cruelty inflicted upon defenceless victims. Anger is expressed at such mistreatments, along with a wish for justice and punishment by fire. It is equally perceptible in Gargantua's vengeful devastation of the Chasteau du Gué du Vede with all those inside. Violence is presented as legitimate and is performed by Folengo's and Rabelais's positive characters in retaliation for undeserved aggression and cruelty, as well as perhaps for resorting to gunpowder. In addition to this, Rabelais introduces an issue that is not problematized in Folengo's mock epic, namely, the impact of violence on those who witness it. How does one react to a scene of violence? If one fights back, as Frère Jean does in the Close of the abbey of Seuilly, and as Ponocrates suggests he would were he king of Paris, how is their violence to be assessed in relation to that of their enemies?

The evolution of artillery and firearms in the late Middle Ages and early modernity changed the way wounding and killing were enacted and pragmatically understood, as well as the way they were ethically justified, and inscribed within prior epistemological traditions regarding embodiment and justice. This development had an impact on medicine as well, since new types of wounds required new forms of cure and medical care—when possible at all.[16] The French military surgeon Ambroise Paré played a decisive role in this respect.[17] Paré published his treatise on wounds in 1551 and began his address to King Henry II with a description of firearms.[18] His comments are unambiguous: firearms are utterly devastating. The development of surgery was urgent and had to be concurrent with that of warfare.

Most notably, the changes caused by the advent of firearms had an impact on the way embodiment was experienced, as well as imagined, fictionalized and fantasized. Literature is a key source of evidence for such an evolution, which is particularly notable in descriptions of fights and wounds, as the latter enact the type of embodiment and kinesis that made sense to authors and readers. We saw that Murrin situates the transitional period at stake between 1440 and 1530.[19] With *Gargantua*, Rabelais stands at the end of this historical period, while another text, *The Alliterative Morte Arthure*, dated to the beginning of Murrin's temporal span, is instrumental to understanding the paradigm shift caused by the use of gunpowder.[20] This strikingly violent text offers numerous descriptions of wounds as they are being inflicted, of projected missiles that predate the gunpowder revolution, and of an aristocratic attitude that is still liable to scorn common fate in the face of catapulted or projected missiles.[21] Passages from this fifteenth-century epic poem will help us assess the mutation manifest in Folengo and Rabelais.

In the *Alliterative Morte Arthure*, as in other medieval epics or romances, a wound typically perforates the body and exposes its inner organs.[22] A knight levels his lance, rides at full speed against his opponent, and spikes him "through the small ribs a span above the waist/so steel plate and spleen were skewered on the spear" ["Aboven the spayre a span, among the short ribbes,/That the splent and the spleen on the spere lenges"; 2060–61].[23] The wounding gesture is located with precision. It pierces the body all the way through an inner organ, the spleen, which remains stuck on the spear. The blood then spills out from a victim whose general shape is preserved despite an imminent death. The body is not dismantled. The blood runs out and even sprays out when the horse leaps forward ["The blood sprent out and spredde as the horse springes"; 2062], but the body remains whole enough finally to fall onto the ground.

It is not rare for opponents to talk to each other before fighting, either simply to provoke the confrontation or also to perform a coded exchange of insults called flyting. In terms of proxemics, it means that the adversaries are close enough to do so: they are, if not at speaking distance, at least at yelling distance. In a passage depicting a duel, Sir Gawain asks his adversary to quit boasting, before they start duelling. They begin by exchanging words, before doing their best to kill each other. Once silent, they level their lances, spur their steeds at full speed, and strike:

> Coupen at aunter by craftes of armes
> Til both the cruel speres brusten at ones;
> Through sheldes they shot and sheered through mailes
> Both sheer through shoulders a shaft-monde large. (2543–46)
>
> [striking freely with all the strength they could summon/until both spear shafts shuddered and shattered;/through shields they shot and sheered through chain mail,/spiking shoulders to the depth of a span.]

Duelling in this passage conforms to typical medieval representations of jousting: opponents ride against each other and strike when close enough to use held lances and wielded swords. Their weapons may burst at the shock, but not their bodies.

Moreover, the distance separating the knights cannot exceed the length of their weapons. Throughout the Middle Ages the implicit rule is very clear: the closer the nobler. The Old English verb *sceotan*, to become Middle English *shoten*, used in "Through sheldes they shot" (2545), does not mean that the knights hurl their spear, but rather that they thrust them through their adversary's shield, and press them further into the chain mails until the spears penetrate deeply into their respective shoulders. When they resort to swords, they strike ("Full stoutly they strike"; 2553) and stab at each other's stomach with steel points ("Stokes at the stomach with steelen pointes"; 2554).

Even in scenes of slaughter and stampede, embodiment implies the preservation of a general corporeal bulk:

> Woundes of wale men workand sides,
> Faces fetteled unfair in feltered lockes
> All craysed, for-trodden with trapped steedes,
> The fairest on folde that figured was ever,
> As fer as a furlong, a thousand at ones! (2148–52)

> [Admirable men, all maimed and mauled,/filthy hair framing once-fair features (faces),/were trodden and trampled by horses in their trappings,/the fairest on earth that were ever formed;/for as far a furlong a thousand lay felled].

In this massacre, dying adversaries cover the ground, but are nevertheless left with a face: "Faces fetteled unfair in feltered lockes" (2149). Bodies are trodden and trampled, and that very fact suggests that they still exist as some kind of whole after the moment of death.

This was less likely to be the case after a gunpowder explosion. The imagination of an early sixteenth-century writer such as Folengo has adjusted to an increased probability of bodily radical dismemberment in combat, as is evidenced by the way he fictionalizes corporeal destruction. In the *Alliterative Morte Arthure*, violence is pervasive and frighteningly graphic, but gunpowder has not yet modified literary representations of warfare: knights clash and strike at each other in close contact with swords and wielded spears. They suffer atrocious injuries, sometimes cleaving a body in two or plunging a blade into an enemy's face, but they are not shattered into shreds of flesh. If they throw missiles, it is from siege engines that hit and smash targets. Mechanics are involved, not powder and firepower. A final passage from the *Alliterative Morte Arthure* shows the implications of such a distinction.

Arthur is besieging the city of Metz in Lorraine. He begins by looking for the best locations to set up siege engines intended to damage the city's protective walls and inner buildings. Inspecting the fortress, he walks by its walls without armour or shield, despite a rain of arbalesters' shots aimed at him ("Allblawsters at Arthur egerly shootes"; 2426). Arthur deems it impossible for commoners' crossbow bolts to wound the anointed king that he is: the "King shrugged off those shafts" ("The king shunt for no shot"; 2428). The plot here condones this fictional assumption, notwithstanding the fact that it draws attention to the near insanity of such an act of bravery: "'Sir,' said Ferrar, 'you flirt with folly ("a folly thou workes")/ in nearing those walls so noticeably noble, ("thus naked in thy noblay")/ coming singly to the city suited only in a surcoat'" (2432–34). After ridiculing the fear of his knight, Arthur claims that the crossbowmen may "win no worship of me" (2444): they will soon lack bolts and arrows, for "Shall never harlot have happe through help of my Lord,/To kill a crowned king with crimson annointed" ("My Lord would not allow any knave to have luck/in killing a crowned king with chrism anointed";

2446–2447). Siege engines and the kind of damage they cause have not yet changed the imagination of writers and their audience.

Such a scene could be written in the England of 1400–1440, despite the use of cannons since the fourteenth century.[24] Mentalities and fiction have not yet shifted to what may be found in Folengo's macaronic epic.[25] *Baldo* was written during the Great Italian Wars, when gunpowder was becoming paramount in the logistics of combat and in the way warfare was conceived. Anointed or not, an aristocrat would be less and less likely to pose as being immune to commoners' bolts and arrows.[26] Indeed, leaders progressively came to stay out of the battlefield to control their tactics from afar, when traditionally they were expected to fight in the middle of the fray.

Folengo and Adam's Apple

In 1517, Folengo wrote a macaronic epic that extended fictionality to new frontiers.[27] In Book 19, Baldo battles against 600,000 armed devils (l. 272). He fights with a contact weapon: his sword. "So the valorous spirit of the heroic Baldo suddenly awakens, and drawing on the fierce courage in his heart, he rushes into the middle of the devils with his sword gleaming" ("brando rutilante," l. 267). He strikes on all sides, while the devils stab him "with hoes and pitchforks and pliers, hooks, grapnels, flaming claws and horns, and scratch and jab him with their horns" (ll. 289–91). But the "might of the Baldensian sword arm strikes like lightning, with thrusts, slashes and various battle strokes" ["Fulminat ensigero Baldensis forcia brazzo/et cum mandrittis, et cum fendentibus, et cum/diversis Guerra tractis"] (ll. 317–19). The hero performs typical chivalric gestures of close combat.

Particular moves are then described. Baldo slays the devil named Malatasca, "whose corpse runs about here and there without its innards ("absque corada"; l. 379), carrying its head which Baldo had lopped off" (378–80).[28] Baldo grabs another devil, Malacoda, "by the tail and swings him around like a sling. Then opening his fist, he releases him into the air ("inde manum slargans hunc lassat abire per auras" l. 383), and off he goes to fall down eight miles away" (ll. 381–4). Three devils try to flee, until "Malabolgia lugs a bag heavy with round cannonballs, and the blackguard launches tough nuts" ("Ecce gravem tundis bolzam Malabolza balottis/baiulat et lanzat crudas boiazza nosellas"; ll. 387–8). These descriptions present a gradation from using a sword in order to perforate and eviscerate, to throwing a body away from one's bare hands, and finally to hurling cannonballs. This last operation is performed by a devil named "Bad-Cannonballs" *Malabolza*, and it triggers the narrator's scandalized reaction:

> Non tamen ad Baldum timidus manigoldus acostat;
> sat sibi quod feriat nec non lontanus amazzet,
> ut nunc qui schioppos, ut nunc qui tempore guerrae
> archibusa ferunt, moschettos paraque moscas. (II. XIX, 387–92)
>
> [But the cowardly rapscallion doesn't go near Baldo; he is content to wound and kill from a distance, like those who nowadays carry rifles and during wartime carry harquebuses, muskets and "fly-swatters"].

Then follows the canonical attack against firearms:

> Isn't it true that any knave, any lice-ridden, greasy scullery-boy, any bread thief hiding behind a wall, watching quietly, taking aim from afar and squeezing the trigger with a rogue hand that should be cut off, can make "toof, taff" echo through the air. Such a one will kill you all by himself and penetrate your chest all by himself—even yours, O most stalwart Giovanni delle Bande Nere of the Medici clan, whose tremendous strength is known throughout the world! (ll. 393–400)

The narrator thus comments on this outrageous mode of modern killing, then listing contemporary figures unfairly killed in this way.

This outburst is followed immediately in the text by a remarkable event. Bombs launched by a flying adversary are imagined. Pragmatically impossible at the time, what will become only too real in the twentieth century after the inception of aeronautical warfare is here conceptualized in a sixteenth-century context via fictionalizing acts.[29]

> Sic Malabolza procul, nunc sub, nunc supra volando
> dardeggiat valido pomranzia ferrea brazzo,
> quae tam praecipiti mandantur fulgure Baldo,
> quam si bombardis ruerent scoccantibus arcem. (vv. 410–13)
>
> [And so Malabolgia from a distance, flying now low, now high, hurls iron oranges with his robust arm, which are fired off at Baldo with lightning speed, like bombards destroying a fortress.]

Whereas the lightning simile was originally used to qualify Baldo's sword, it is now associated with cannonballs.

On the one hand, Malabolgia adopts the typical distance of the coward who shoots from a safe position. But, on the other, he can maximize the use of cannonballs since he is able to fly, being a supernatural creature. He may even adjust his height and shoot from the right altitude. The concrete and the imaginary intermingle to produce unexpected configurations.[30] The latter are staged in the highly and ever fictional framework of a battle against devils, semi-parodic of a long European cultural and religious tradition, whose double literary apex are Dante's *Divine Comedy* in the Middle Ages, and Milton's *Paradise Lost* in the modern era.

In Folengo, the biblical tradition is invested with new fictional possibilities. Baldo reacts promptly to the shooting. In order to protect himself, he shrewdly grabs Beelzebub and turns him into a shield, thus warding off Malabolgia's cannonballs. While impacted by the missiles, Beelzebub remains whole for some time. Malabolgia is ordered by other devils to stop firing, because Beelzebub is "foremost leader and arch-devil":

> However, Malabolgia pays no attention at all to such an order and instead takes up the apple with which he had once felled Adam [capit pomum, quo quondam stravit Adamum; l. 439] and throws an apple-bomb [*pomatamque tirat*, l. 440], not like those usually fired by Neapolitan youths, but like those from a Milanese cannon, a culverin (sed quam colubrine Milani; l. 441). It screams as it flies by, and its flame sheds light. (ll. 438–42)

Beelzebub is hit by the apple and "feels two of his ribs break" (l. 444). The whole army turns in anger against Malabolgia, but Baldo helps him. He "puts his sword back in its sheath, with both hands he grabs Beelzebub by the feet" and starts swinging his body down onto the devil's own soldiers, lacerating him on the latter's horns, pitchforks and hooks (ll. 445–54). It will be the hero's thrashing and slashing movements that ultimately will prove most efficient, not the shooting and bombing gestures of the devil.

A dissention in the army ensues and the devils stop harassing Baldo with pitchforks and cannonballs ("seu forchis sive balottis"; l. 494). Baldo "has nothing in his hands to fight with any longer; in fact, his sword rests in its sheath and does not want to leave it" (ll. 496–497). We are next told why Baldo finds himself empty-handed. "After an hour of serving as a club, Beelzebub is reduced to 170,000 bite-size pieces; only one of his goosefeet remained in Baldo's hand, but some of his parts, like the spleen, the offal and the intestines, hang from trees; the rest were minced into tiny particles by Baldo's arm ("per Baldi brazzum tridefacta minutim"; l. 503) and sprayed onto the black face of each devil ("aspersere nigram faciem cuiusque diabli"; l. 504)" (ll. 498–504). Then Beelzebub "went looking for fragments of his body parts" ("ibat membrorum quaerens fragmenta suorum") (ll. 505–506). At this stage, the narrator makes a comment that evinces all the potentials of human imagination and capacity for fictionalizing acts.

> Certamenter habet pro doia plangere causam
> sed quae membra sibi doleant nessuna trovantur,
> non qui bagnentur pietosis fletibus occhi,
> non quae lingua cridet magnis urlatibus 'Oyme',
> non qui cum gemitu tampellent pectora pugni. (ll. 507–511)
>
> [He certainly has good cause to cry in pain, but the parts that could weep for him cannot be found. There are no eyes that might moisten with piteous tears; no tongue which might cry out, "Woe is me!" in loud shrieks; no fists which might hammer at a chest with a hollow sound].

The victim has lost his face. He is looking for his face and, thereby, for the facial organs (eyes and tongue) that would enable him to cry, scream, and vent his distress. The rest of his body is equally concerned by his search, as he is looking (without eyes or hands) for his fists and chest, wishing to bang his torso to further express his pangs at being disembodied—an ultimate kinesic paradox. Folengo's fictionalization of disembodiment (even more radical than dismemberment) is both remarkably original and eminently situated within history. Kinesic analysis is a way of acknowledging such originality and historical situatedness. To address the above passage, readers resort to their kinesic intelligence, whereby they make sense of all manner of possible and impossible movements and actions, including disembodiment, while they also situate these very movements in a context that provides an orientation to their interpretive efforts and the type of inferences the text may lead them to adduce.[31]

The fact that Baldo uses his hands only, not even his sword, is stressed. He fights in close contact, notwithstanding his adversaries' supernatural nature. Meanwhile, direct contact with him results in the type of disintegration cannonballs and firearms produce, suggesting that the superhero has the same impact artillery does. His heroism is able to produce the results afforded by new technologies. Novel modes of killing affect the relation to embodiment and the way this relation feeds the imagination—for better or for worse. Notably, in this passage, Adam's Edenic apple is reinvested in unprecedented ways. The formal analogy between apple and cannonball provides a link between destruction as narrated in Genesis (the Fall and the origin of doom) and destruction as imagined in Book 19 of *Baldo*. In the latter, to destroy is to use the same traditional key object or affordance, the biblical apple, loaded with symbolic implications of catastrophe, but with a gesture that differs radically. From transgression by ingestion and incorporation, Adam's apple becomes a projectile wherewith to shoot one's enemy. The act of transgression looks like the latest available technological development. As such it benefits from the positive qualification of lightning, usually saved for divine or semi-divine attributes. Adam's apple in Folengo and, as we now shall see, the shaft of the Cross in Rabelais are similarly reinvested with new meanings and functions.

Rabelais and the Shaft of the Cross

In Rabelais, Frère Jean, a Benedictine monk of the abbey of Seuilly, slaughters soldiers intent on sacking the place. He does so in close contact and by means of the shaft of a Cross. He even impales them with it: "Sy quelq'un gravoyt en une arbre pensant y estre en seureté, icelluy de son baston empaloyt par le fondement" (80) ["If any one clambered into a tree and thought he was safe up there he impaled him with his shaft through the fundament"] (295). Whether with Adam's apple or the shaft of the Christian cross, such use of symbolically charged objects calls for attention. Admittedly, Frère Jean does not use the Cross itself but the staff that supports it. Still, it is not any kind of staff: by being defined in its association with the Cross, it connects the latter to Frère Jean's action.

The abbey of Seuilly is attacked and pillaged by troops belonging to Picrochole, a king who wages war by means of all kinds of artillery.

> [F]eut par son esdict constitué le seigneur Grippeminaud sus l'avantgarde, en laquelle feurent contez seize mille hacquebutiers, vingt cinq mille avanturiers. À l'artillerie fut commis le grand escuyer Toucquedillon, en laquelle feurent contées neuf cens quatorze grosses pieces de bronze, en canons, double canons, baselicz, serpentines, coulevrines, bombardes, faulcons, passevolans, spiroles, et aultres pieces. (76)

> [By his edict the Seigneur de Grippeminaud was placed in the vanguard, which comprised sixteen thousand men armed with harquebuses and

> twenty-five thousand soldiers of fortune. The ordnance was entrusted to Toucquedillon, the Grand Equerry; in which were counted nine hundred and fourteen great bronze guns: cannons, cannon-royals, basilisks, serpentines, culverins, bombards, falcons, passé-volants, falconets and other field-pieces]. (291)

The reader is thereby reminded of artillery in all its forms, shortly before Frère Jean's great act of slaughter in the Close of the abbey.

After Picrochole's troops have reached and savagely plundered the town of Seuilly, the main part of the army departs, leaving behind a few hundred men, who break into the Close of Frère Jean's abbey to waste, spoil and steal. The monks are helpless. Seeing their source of wine threatened, Frère Jean decides to take action. He grabs the shaft of the Cross, which is concrete, made of the heart of a cornel-tree, and said to be as long as a lance ("long comme une lance"). Just like a lance, it impacts bodies quite directly, Frère Jean striking in the old fencing style, that is, indiscriminately: "frapant à tors et à travers à vieille escrime" (79). Despite its lance-like length, Frère Jean does not throw, propel or hurl his recycled weapon. With it, he smashes, thrashes, strikes, thrusts, hits, breaks and the like.

> In some cases he battered their brains out ["es uns escarbouilloyt la cervelle"]; in others, he fractured their arms and legs ["es aultres rompoyt bras et jambes"]; in others, he dislocated the vertebrae of the neck ["es aultres deslochoyt les spondyles du coul"]; and in others, he ruptured the kidneys ["es aultres demoulloyt les reins"], bashed in their noses ["avalloyt le nez"], blacked their eyes ["poschoyt les yeulx"], smashed their mandibles ["fendoyt les mandibules"], knocked their teeth down their throats ["enfonçoyt les dens en la gueule"], stove in their shoulder-blades ["descroulloyt les omoplates"], gangrened their legs ["sphaceloyt les greves"], dislocated their thighs ["desgondoyt les ischies"] and splintered their fore-arms ["debezilloit les fauciles"]. (295)[32]

Through anatomical specification, Rabelais describes wounds that smack of both Homeric and medieval epics. Meanwhile, the very listing of the wounds is less common and suggests thorough dismantling, where each victim adds to an overall fictional body torn to pieces. Ultimately, the general impression is that of slaughter by explosion owing to the fast succession of radical strokes. Only here, the explosion is that of Frère Jean's vengeful energy, not the blast caused by the ignition of gunpowder. Gargantua a few pages later will have the same—albeit less detailed—devastating impact on Picrochole's army in the Chasteau du Gué du Vede. Frère Jean and Gargantua are in this sense comparable to Baldo, who shatters Beelzebub to pieces.

Florence Weinberg spells out the problem that Frère Jean's massacre poses to critics: "Thus, in order to protect Rabelais' honour for the twentieth-century reader, we try to avoid the accusation of sadism. How to explain that Rabelais created this merry murderer? That he enjoyed so much the surgical depiction of a barbarous violence?"[33] Weinberg offers an answer to this by way of an allegorical and anagogical reading: "Those who ransack the vineyard represent the enemies of the true faith," namely, "any group separated from the spirit of the true Christianity and the Evangelical Church. [...] Jean defends the vineyard, source of the wine that symbolizes the essence of Christianity. [...] He is situated on an anagogical and allegorical level, as *co-operator of God*."[34] In order to spare Rabelais from the accusation of sadism, Weinberg makes a fundamentalist out of him, who would be happy to kill in the name of his faith as long as a symbolic rationale might allow it.[35] But if such is the case, then what is the point of Rabelais's anatomical precision? Is it enough to think that the doctor in him yielded to scientific temptation? And how are we to account for the cynical reference in the text to murdered women and children, the "usual" collateral victims of wars and massacres? (297).

In *L'Esthétique de Rabelais*, Demerson offers a different perspective. He reads in Frère Jean's violence a way to call into question "typically epic values." [...] "Indeed, in him (Jean), Rabelais evinces that which constitutes the spirit of epics: presumption and cruelty. Frère Jean's epic has the frenzied rhythm, the joyful cruelty of classical and modern heroic poems. [...] Such horrors find their source in Homer, as well as Virgil."[36] In her essay, Weinberg argues against Demerson's reading: "Demerson invents a Jean who is to be reprimanded, in contrast to a Rabelais who slyly condemns the savage values of epic songs."[37] The contrast between Weinberg's and Demerson's interpretations suggests that Rabelais succeeded in raising the problem of violence. Violence was, is, and remains, a problem. To try and offer a palatable solution (Evangelic or parodic) to the slaughter episode might be missing Rabelais's point.

An alternative approach may be to focus on kinesic information *per se* and grapple with the specific function violence has in a given text. Indeed, wounds in Homer's *Iliad*, in Virgil's *Aeneid*, and in Rabelais's *Gargantua* serve entirely different purposes. For one thing, they are the expression of distinct logics of embodiment, and they cannot be reduced to anachronistic notions of cruelty.[38] Rabelais conveys Frère Jean's action via the extensive repetition of kinesic verbs of physical impact, emphasizing dismantling by contact. This aspect of the text addresses one central problem in the advent of firearms, topical at the time, that is, the anonymity of the killer. In the Close of Seuilly, violence has a name. Not so when one is shot from afar. Frère Jean has a face, it is even "bien fendu de gueule" (78) ["loud-mouthed"] (293). Such a blunt endorsement of agency has an assertive quality that becomes highly significant if we place it in the context of the gunpowder revolution. Thus, the point might possibly not be symbolic via anagogy, or ethical via parody. Rather, it would be literal and kinesic. It answers the question of agency by giving a face to he who strikes. It is not meant to reduce the horror of violence, quite the contrary. It is a way of calling it by its name: a human destroying other humans. The wound remains open. Rabelais is not trying to reduce the fracture. He lexically performs the de-anatomization of bodies into smithereens.

In her introduction to Ambroise Paré's *Treatise on Wounds*, Marie-Madeleine Fragonard highlights the modernity of Paré's efforts. He was a surgeon, not a learned doctor trained in Hippocratic and Galenic theories. The horror of firearm wounds prompted him, like other surgeons before and after him, to find concrete and straightforward solutions to new injuries, "sans caution d'autorité et sans latin!" [without the backing of authorities nor Latin!][39] Paré wanted urgently to teach the remedies he had discovered. Before him, Rabelais, a trained doctor, writes a literature for the people, whether bishops or "vérolés" (5) ["pox-ridden patients"], with extensive references to European culture and knowledge, as a humanist who could read Latin and Greek, and was versed in all manner of French dialects. Yet, despite this distinction, Rabelais, just like Paré, was surely faced with the wounded bodies that covered the battlefields of his time. He may thus have tried to come to terms with acts of mass violence, both as doctor and writer. In the slaughter passage, by means of literature, Rabelais lexically spells out the wounding impact of cannon shooting. In verbal proliferation, each carefully selected medical and anatomical term participates in a scene, where Frère Jean's explosive action makes us imagine and conceptualize the multiple moments that constitute the radical and sudden disintegration of human bodies.[40]

Ellen Spolsky explains that "the prevailing contracts of fiction guide us in exercising our innate abilities to move between types and tokens, both concrete images and abstract concepts being open sets."[41] Rabelais with his cross and Folengo with his apple fired like a cannonball produce fictional acts, which lead us to exercise our cognitive and intellective "abilities to move between types"—say, a kinesic distinction between shooting and striking—"and tokens"—say, Folengo's apple and Rabelais's cross—"both concrete images and abstract concepts being open sets."[42] Via such open sets, or levers of productive indeterminacy, literature sets the mind open and invents new ways of relating to a novel reality, via writers' and readers' cognitive acts grounded in kinesic intelligence and imagination. By focusing on concrete historical aspects in order then to adduce possible kinesic inferences from the texts, I hope to have shown how an enhanced attention to kinesis in literary analysis may shed light on challenging fictional gestures, expressive of complex connections between historical facts and the imaginary power of literature.

Notes

1. Teofilo Folengo used the pseudonym Merlin Coccaie. Ann Mullaney writes in her introduction to her translation of Folengo's *Baldo*, "Folengo clearly reached a large public. One enthusiastic reader was François Rabelais (1494–1553), also a one-time Benedictine monk, who borrowed episodes from *Baldo* and adapted many of Folengo's traits, such as his predilection for synonyms, his use of long lists and fictional authorities, his occasional intromission of the authorial "I," and his devotion to the bottle."; see Teofilo Folengo, *Baldo*, trans. Ann E. Mullaney (Cambridge MA: Harvard University Press, 2007), 2:vii. A French translation of *Baldo* was published in 1606 as the *Histoire macaronique de Merlin Coccaie, prototype de Rablais* [sic], signalling in its title Folengo's influence on Rabelais. A well-known borrowing is the episode of Panurge and the sheep. Also, "the French writer honours Folengo by placing him last on the long list of books in the Library of St. Victor: *Merlinus Coccaius, De patria diabolorum* (Merlin Cocaio, On the Devil's Country), right after *Antidotarum animae* (Antidotes for the Soul)"; see Folengo, *Baldo*, trans. Mullaney, 1:xviii. The first edition of *Baldo* came out in 1517 and the last in 1552, several years after Folengo's death in 1544. Mullaney uses Mario Chiesa's edition for her translation, which I cite throughout this essay; Teofilo Folengo, *Baldus*, ed. Mario Chiesa, and trans. Gérard Genot and Paul Larivaille (Paris: Les Belles Lettres, 2007).

   On Folengo's artistic endeavour and style in his fascinating mix of Latin and dialectal Italian, a linguistic cookery that explains the name macaronic, formed on the name of the Italian pasta *macaroni*, see Michel Jeanneret, *Des mets et des mots: banquets et propos de table à la Renaissance* (Paris: José Corti, 1987), 202–3. See also Marcel Tetel, "Rabelais et Folengo,"

Comparative Literature 15, no. 4 (1963): 357–64; A. E. B. Coldiron, "Macaronic Verse, Plurilingual Printing, and the Uses of Translation," in *Early Modern Cultures of Translation*, ed. Karen Newman and Jane Tylus (Philadelphia: University of Pennsylvania Press, 2015), 56–75; Barbara C. Bowen, "Rabelais and Folengo Once Again," in *Rabelais in Context. Proceedings of the 1991 Vanderbilt Conference*, ed. Barbara C. Bowen (Birmingham, AL: Summa Publications, 1993), 207–31.
2. See Geoffrey Parker, "The Gunpowder Revolution," in *The Cambridge History of Warfare*, ed. Geoffrey Parker (Cambridge: Cambridge University Press, 2005), 101–14.
3. Ellen Spolsky, "Elaborated Knowledge: Reading Kinesis in Pictures," *Poetics Today* 17, no. 2 (1996): 158–9.
4. My focus is on kinesis and the gunpowder revolution. Therefore I will not discuss the status of religious symbols in the Reformation.
5. J. R. Hale, *War and Society in Renaissance Europe 1450–1620* (Leicester: Leicester University Press and Fontana Press, 1985), 46. "Gunpowder consists of three ingredients—saltpeter, sulphur, and charcoal—the best proportions being approximately 75% saltpetre, 10% sulphur, and 15% charcoal."; see Kelly Devries and Robert Douglas Smith, *Medieval Military Technology* (Toronto: University of Toronto Press, 2012), 152.
6. Michael Murrin, *History and Warfare in Renaissance Epic* (Chicago: The University of Chicago Press, 1994), 123.
7. Murrin, *History and Warfare in Renaissance Epic*, 123.
8. Regarding Ariosto, complexity and tension are also perceptible, but extra-textually. Indeed, Ariosto's patron, Alfonso d'Este, was famously keen on developing artillery, and "gained a European-wide reputation as an innovator in the manufacture of powder." His "court of Ferrara was always among the leaders in the arm race"; see Dave Henderson, "Power Unparalleled: Gunpowder Weapons and the Early *Furioso*," *Shifanoia* 13–14 (1992): 110, 116. Piero Floriani calls Alfonso d'Este "l'un des plus grands artilleurs de son temps"; see his "Guerre et chevaliers 'avec reproche' dans le *Roland Furieux*," in *L'Homme de guerre au XVIe siècle*, ed. Gabriel-André Pérouse, André Thierry and André Tournon (Saint-Etienne: Publications de l'Université de Saint-Etienne, 1992), 298.
9. Michael Murrin, *History and Warfare*, 125.
10. Murrin, *History and Warfare*, 125.
11. Murrin, *History and Warfare*, 128.
12. DeVries and Smith, *Medieval Military Technology*, 144–45.
13. Maurice Keen "The Changing Scene: Guns, Gunpowder, and Permanent Armies," in *Medieval Warfare: A History*, ed. Maurice Keen (Oxford: Oxford University Press, 1999), 280.
14. DeVries and Smith, *Medieval Military Technology*, 156.

15. François Rabelais, *Œuvres complètes*, ed. Mireille Huchon (Paris: Gallimard, 1994), 101; François Rabelais, *Gargantua and Pantagruel*, trans. M. A. Screech (London: Penguin Classics, 2006), 318. All subsequent references are to this edition and translation are supplied in parentheses.
16. DeVries explains that "It was not until 1460 that any surgical manual even mentions gunshot wounds, and it was even later before these wounds are given specific and distinct treatment in surgical writings."; Kelly DeVries, "Military Surgical Practice and the Advent of Gunpowder Weaponry," *Canadian Bulletin of Medical History* 7 (1990): 133.
17. "In 1536, at the siege of Turin, French military surgeon Ambroise Paré changed surgical history. At that time, it was the custom to treat gunshot wounds by pouring boiling oil into them, often without removing the fragment or bullet. Paré, having run out of this cauterizing mixture, was forced to use a non-abrasive digestive to treat some of his wounded patients. This surgical procedure ultimately proved that gunshot wounds should not be treated by cauterization. Gunpowder weapons, however, had been in use for more than two centuries before Paré's discovery"; see DeVries, "Military Surgical Practice": 131. See also Jean Céard, "La médecine de l'homme de guerre à la Renaissance," in *L'Homme de guerre au XVIe siècle*, ed. Gabriel-André Pérouse, André Thierry and André Tournon (Saint-Etienne: Publications de l'Université de Saint-Etienne, 1992), 229–40.
18. Ambroise Paré, *La manière de traiter les plaies*, ed. Marie-Madeleine Fragonard (Paris: Presses Universitaires de France et Genève, 2007), fol. aa ii.
19. Murrin, *History and Warfare in Renaissance Epic*, 123.
20. Lee Patterson, *Negotiating the Past: The Historical Understanding of Medieval Literature* (Madison: The University of Wisconsin Press, 1987), 212: "The poem survives in a single manuscript of about 1440, but was probably composed in the form in which we now have it about forty years earlier." ... "The manuscript is Lincoln Cathedral MS91, written by Robert Thornton," hence called the Lincoln Thornton. It is even likely that the poem was "composed over a considerable period of time, through a process of accretion and revision familiar to medieval literature, and that it embodies a kind of historical layering, with level laid on level."
21. Hale, "Gunpowder and the Renaissance," 120: "The chivalrous contempt for firearms as a coward's weapon had been anticipated by a scorn for missile weapons that went back to the Greeks." Hale provides examples from Euripides and from various early modern texts written in Italy, France, Germany, Spain and England. Guns were deemed both cowardly and devilish. However, opinions were more nuanced in England, owing to the crucial role played by longbows in the Hundred Years War. "English pride in her missile troops, the archers, meant that while Englishmen could

condemn guns as being devilish or deride them as inefficient, few thought of them as cowardly" (122). See also Evelyn Tribble, "Where are the Archers in Shakespeare?" *ELH* 82 (2015): 789–814.

22. On this logic of embodiment, see Guillemette Bolens, "La momification dans la littérature médiévale: L'embaumement d'Hector chez Benoît de Sainte-Maure, Guido delle Colonne et John Lydgate," in "La pelle umana/The Human Skin," ed. Agostino Paravicini Bagliani, special issue, *Micrologus* 13: 213–311; Guillemette Bolens, *La Logique du corps articulaire: Les articulations du corps humain dans la littérature occidentale* (Rennes: Presses Universitaires de Rennes, 2007), "Introduction."
23. *The Alliterative Morte Arthure: The Death of King Arthur*, trans. Simon Armitage (New York: W. W. Norton & Co, 2012). All references are to this edition, with line numbers supplied in parenthesis.
24. The English king Edward III used cannons "to create noise and panic" in the battle of Crécy during the Hundred Years War and "by 1400 gunpowder weaponry appeared in nearly every engagement of the war"; see DeVries, "Military Surgical Practice," 135.
25. Floriani, "Guerre et chevaliers," 295: "Le développement rapide de l'art de la guerre n'implique pas … un changement aussi rapide des conceptions et des valeurs qui sont liées à la guerre: l'idéologie nobiliaire de l'aristocratie européenne, pour laquelle la valeur individuelle est la seule mesure du jugement militaire, impose encore ses lois." [The rapid development of the art of war does not imply … a correspondingly rapid change in the mentalities and values linked to war: the noble ideology of the European aristocracy, for whom individual value was the sole measure of military judgement, continues to dominate.]
26. DeVries, "Military Surgical Practice," 136: "This interest in gunpowder weaponry increased as the war progressed. As guns became more numerous and more accurate and powerful, more soldiers were killed and wounded. Small guns fired metal balls, usually made of lead or iron, and larger guns fired stone balls, especially fashioned for that purpose. Gunshot wounds from both these weapons could be and were often fatal; metal balls could pierce the skin, while larger stone balls could kill on impact with the body or by splintering into fragments which would then enter the torso or limbs. Sometimes in medieval chronicles these fatalities are unnamed, mostly because of their low station, but on other occasions gunshots killed more prominent victims. In 1383, at the siege of Ypres, a 'very brave English esquire,' Louis Lin, was killed by a cannon shot. In 1414, the Bastard of Bourbon was killed by gunshot at Soisson. In 1438, Don Pedro, the brother of the king of Castille, was decapitated by a gunshot during the siege of Capuana at Naples. […] Finally, in 1460, James II of Scotland died when one of his large cannons exploded next to him. Perhaps the most famous

death by gunshot during the Hundred Years War occurred in 1428 when Thomas Montagu, earl of Salisbury and leader of the English forces in France, 'a worthi werrioure amonge all Cristen men,' was killed at Orleans when a stone cannon ball fired from a bombard (the largest type of siege gun) shattered and mortally wounded him in the head."

27. On Folengo's poetry, see Coldiron, "Macaronic Verse," 56–75.
28. Folengo, ed. Mullaney, 1:xvii: Folengo "borrows and distorts many of the names of Dante's devils." See also Marcel Tetel, "Rabelais et Folengo: *De Patria Diabolorum*," in "Rabelais en son demi-millénaire," ed. Jean Céard and Jean-Claude Margolin, special issue, *Études Rabelaisiennes* 21 (1988): 203–24. One of the devils in Folengo is named Bombarda: i.e. cannon.
29. On fictionalizing acts, see Wolfgang Iser, *The Fictive and the Imaginary: Charting Literary Anthropology* (Baltimore: Johns Hopkins University Press, 1993).
30. Iser, *The Fictive and the Imaginary*; Ellen Spolsky, *The Contracts of Fiction: Cognition, Culture, Community* (Oxford: Oxford University Press, 2015); Ellen Spolsky, "Why and How to Take the Fruit and Leave the Chaff," *SubStance* 30, 1/2 (2001): 177–98.
31. Perceptual simulations are central to the cognitive efforts that ground kinesic intelligence; see Guillemette Bolens, *The Style of Gestures: Embodiment and Cognition in Literary Narrative* (Baltimore: John Hopkins University Press, 2012).
32. For the French original, see Rabelais, *Œuvres complètes*, 79.
33. Florence Weinberg, *Rabelais et les leçons du rire: Paraboles évangéliques et néoplatoniciennes* (Orléans: Paradigme, 2000), 74.
34. Weinberg, *Rabelais et les leçons du rire*, 75.
35. Anthony Russell writes that, "Like Rabelais, Folengo wrote a mock-epic informed by the spirit of evangelical radicalism central to reformist ideology. Both authors, moreover, levelled some of their most savage satire against the absurdities of theological discourse. Both were monks who left their monasteries on account of their heterodox beliefs and who spent much of the remainder of their lives as wanderers, either defending, concealing, or apologizing for those beliefs." Russell further remarks that "the Baldus would have constituted for Rabelais the only example of a fictional work written in the epic mode with an explicit contemporary reform polemic as one of its central motivations." See Anthony Presti Russell, "Epic Agon and the Strategy of Reform in Folengo and Rabelais," *Comparative Literature Studies* 34, no. 2 (1997): 119–48.
36. Guy Demerson, *L'Esthétique de Rabelais* (Paris: Sedes, 1996), 136–37. See also Guy Demerson, "Violence: Humanisme et facétie," *Europe* 757 (1992): 67–79.
37. Weinberg, *Rabelais et les leçons du rire*, 74.

38. In *La Logique du corps articulaire*, I analyse the logic of embodiment that is extant in the *Iliad.* Some aspects of embodiment in Virgil's *Aeneid* are discussed in Guillemette Bolens, "Le corps de la guerrière: Camille dans l'Enéide de Virgile," in *Körperkonzepte/Concepts du corps: Contributions aux études genre interdisciplinaires*, ed. Franziska Frei Gerlach, Annette Kreis-Schinck, Claudia Opitz, Béatrice Ziegler (Münster: Waxmann, 2003), 47–56. For more on the logic of embodiment, see also Guillemette Bolens, "Continuité et transformation des logiques corporelles," *History and Philosophy of the Life Sciences* 25 (2003): 471–80.
39. Paré, *La manière de traiter les plaies*, 11.
40. Jean-Charles Sournia writes of this scene "Bien entendu Rabelais use et abuse de tous les procédés. Il ajoute les spondyles aux vertèbres, alors que vertèbre est un vieux mot français compris de tous, quand spondyle est nouveau et inconnu des lecteurs, d'autres fois il prend un mot pour l'autre" ["Of course Rabelais uses and abuses every trick in the book. He attaches the spondyls to the vertebrae, when in fact 'vertèbre' is an old French word understood by everybody, whereas 'spondyle' is new and unknown to his readers; at other times he uses the one for the other"], "Le vocabulaire médical de Rabelais," in "Rabelais pour le XXIe siècle," ed. Michel Simonin, special issue, *Études Rabelaisiennes* 33 (1998): 293.
41. Spolsky, *Contracts of Fiction*, 18.
42. Spolsky, *Contracts of Fiction*, 18.

Bibliography

(The) Alliterative Morte Arthure: The Death of King Arthur. Translated by Simon Armitage. New York: W. W. Norton & Co, 2012.

Bolens, Guillemette. *La Logique du corps articulaire: Les articulations du corps humain dans la littérature occidentale.* Rennes: Presses Universitaires de Rennes, 2000/2007.

———. Le corps de la guerrière: Camille dans l'*Énéide* de Virgile. In *Körperkonzepte/Concepts du corps: Contributions aux études genre interdisciplinaires*, edited by Franziska Frei Gerlach, Annette Kreis-Schinck, Claudia Opitz, Béatrice Ziegler, 47–56. Münster: Waxmann, 2003a.

———. Continuité et transformation des logiques corporelles. *History and Philosophy of the Life Sciences* 25 (2003b): 471–80.

———. La momification dans la littérature médiévale: L'embaumement d'Hector chez Benoît de Sainte-Maure, Guido delle Colonne et John Lydgate. In *La pelle umana/The Human Skin*, edited by Agostino Paravicini Bagliani. Special issue, *Micrologus* 13 (2005): 213–31.

———. *The Style of Gestures: Embodiment and Cognition in Literary Narrative.* Baltimore: Johns Hopkins University Press, 2012.

Bowen, Barbara C. Rabelais and Folengo Once Again. In *Rabelais in Context. Proceedings of the 1991 Vanderbilt Conference*, edited by Barbara C. Bowen, 207–31. Birmingham, AL: Summa Publications, 1993.

———. Rabelais's Unreadable Books. *Renaissance Quarterly* 48, no. 4 (1995): 742–58.

Céard, Jean. La médicine de l'homme de guerre à la Renaissance. In *L'Homme de guerre au XVIe siècle*, edited by Gabriel-André Pérouse, André Thierry and André Tournon, 229–40. Saint-Etienne: Publications de l'Université de Saint-Etienne, 1992.

Coldiron, A. E. B. Macaronic Verse, Plurilingual Printing, and the Uses of Translation. In *Early Modern Cultures of Translation*, edited by Karen Newman and Jane Tylus, 56–75. Philadelphia: University of Pennsylvania Press, 2015.

Demerson, Guy. Violence: Humanisme et facétie. *Europe* 757 (1992): 67–79.

———. *L'Esthétique de Rabelais*. Paris: Sedes, 1996.

DeVries, Kelly. Military Surgical Practice and the Advent of Gunpowder Weaponry. *Canadian Bulletin of Medical History* 7 (1990): 131–46.

DeVries, Kelly, and Robert Douglas Smith. *Medieval Military Technology*. Toronto: University of Toronto Press, 2012.

Floriani, Piero. Guerre et chevaliers 'avec reproche' dans le *Roland Furieux*. In *L'Homme de guerre au XVIe siècle*, edited by Gabriel-André Pérouse, André Thierry and André Tournon, 289–99. Saint-Etienne: Publications de l'Université de Saint-Etienne, 1992.

Folengo, Teofilo. *Baldo*. Translated by Ann E. Mullaney. 2 vols. Cambridge MA: Harvard University Press, 2007a.

———. *Baldus*. Edited by Mario Chiesa and translated by Gérard Genot and Paul Larivaille. 3 vols. Paris: Les Belles Lettres, 2007b.

Fontaine, Marie Madeleine. Quaresmeprenant: l'image littéraire et la contestation de l'analogie médicale. In *Libertés et savoirs du corps à la Renaissance*, edited by Marie Madeleine Fontaine, 195–220. Caen: Paradigme, 1993.

Hale, J. R. Gunpowder and the Renaissance: An Essay in the History of Ideas. In *From the Renaissance to the Counter-Reformation*, edited by Charles H. Carter, 113–44. London: Jonathan Cape, 1966.

———. *War and Society in Renaissance Europe 1450–1620*. Leicester: Leicester University Press and Fontana Press, 1985.

Hall, Bert S. *Weapons and Warfare in Renaissance Europe: Gunpowder, Technology, and Tactics*. Baltimore: The Johns Hopkins University Press, 1997.

Henderson, Dave. Power Unparalleled: Gunpowder Weapons and the Early *Furioso*. *Shifanoia* 13–14 (1992): 109–31.

Iser, Wolfgang. *The Fictive and the Imaginary: Charting Literary Anthropology*. Baltimore: Johns Hopkins University Press, 1993.

Jeanneret, Michel. *Des mets et des mots: Banquets et propos de table à la Renaissance*. Paris: José Corti, 1987.

Keen, Maurice. The Changing Scene: Guns, Gunpowder, and Permanent Armies. In *Medieval Warfare: A History*, edited by Maurice Keen, 273–91. Oxford: Oxford University Press, 1999.

Murrin, Michael. *History and Warfare in Renaissance Epic*. Chicago: The University of Chicago Press, 1994.

Paré, Ambroise. *La manière de traiter les plaies*. Edited by Marie-Madeleine Fragonard. Paris: Presses Universitaires de France, 2007.

Parker, Geoffrey. *The Military Revolution: Military Innovation and the Rise of the West: 1500–1800*. Cambridge: Cambridge University Press, 1990.

———. The Gunpowder Revolution. In *The Cambridge History of Warfare*, edited by Geoffrey Parker, 101–14. Cambridge: Cambridge University Press, 2005.

Patterson, Lee. *Negotiating the Past: The Historical Understanding of Medieval Literature*. Madison: The University of Wisconsin Press, 1987.

Rabelais, François. *Œuvres complètes*. Edited by Mireille Huchon. Paris: Gallimard, 1994.

———. *Gargantua and Pantagruel*. Translated by M. A. Screech. London: Penguin Classics, 2006.

Russell, Anthony Presti. Epic Agon and the Strategy of Reform in Folengo and Rabelais. *Comparative Literature Studies* 34, no. 2 (1997): 119–48.

Sournia, Jean-Charles. Le vocabulaire médical de Rabelais. In *Rabelais pour le XXIe siècle*, edited by Michel Simonin. Special Issue, *Études Rabelaisiennes* 33 (1998): 291–97.

Spolsky, Ellen. Elaborated Knowledge: Reading Kinesis in Pictures. *Poetics Today* 17, no. 2 (1996): 157–80.

———. Why and How to Take the Fruit and Leave the Chaff. In *On the Origin of Fictions: Interdisciplinary Perspectives*. Special Issue, *SubStance* 30, no. 1/2 (2001): 177–98.

———. *The Contracts of Fiction: Cognition, Culture, Community*. Oxford: Oxford University Press, 2015.

Tetel, Marcel. Rabelais et Folengo. *Comparative Literature* 15, no. 4 (1963): 357–64.

———. Rabelais et Folengo. *De Patria Diabolorum*. In *Rabelais en son demi-millénaire*, edited by Jean Céard and Jean-Claude Margolin. Special Issue, *Études Rabelaisiennes* 21 (1988): 203–24.

Tribble, Evelyn. Where are the Archers in Shakespeare? *ELH* 82 (2015): 789–814.

Weinberg, Florence. *Rabelais et les leçons du rire: Paraboles évangéliques et néoplatoniciennes*. Orléans: Paradigme, 2000.

CHAPTER 7

The Finger in the Eye: Jacques Duval's *Traité des Hermaphrodits* (1612)

Dominique Brancher

In her innovative work on the "style of gestures," Guillemette Bolens draws on contributions from the cognitive sciences as a basis for her hypothesis that a work generates "perceptual simulations" in its readers. The crucial point is this: this mental stratagem has the same effect on the perceptual activity of the body as if the action had *actually* been carried out.[1] Contrary to a rhetoric of figures whose master form is hypotyposis—and which makes *ut pictura poesis* its motto—reading is thus not merely *seeing*:

> Reading does not place us in front of paintings, but rather involves us in plurimodal operations, visual—tactile—acoustic, sometimes olfactory, gustatory, always intellectual and sensory-motor, emotional and conceptual […].[2]

Parts of this article are elaborated in Dominique Brancher, *Equivoques de la pudeur. Fabrique d'une passion à la Renaissance* (Geneva: Droz, 2015).

D. Brancher (✉)
Basel University, Basel, Switzerland

K. Banks, T. Chesters (eds.), *Movement in Renaissance Literature*, Cognitive Studies in Literature and Performance,
https://doi.org/10.1007/978-3-319-69200-5_7

Reading is therefore not an activity purely of the mind, which frees one from one's corporeal reality, but a commitment that mobilizes all the instruments of the mind and of perception, thereby challenging a long dominant dualism. The act of reading is rooted in corporeality, a fact long exploited by erotic literature of the kind "read with only one hand."[3] It choreographs sexual ballets, and induces its reader to perform them again inwardly, with a perceptual intensity that comes close to that of a real embrace.

In his enthusiastic review of Bolens's work, François Vanoosthuyse underlines the unique role of the "notion of corporeality" and of kinesic play in erotic literature, where the text shows something that the brain or indeed the body repeats.[4] A fitting example of this is the sensual action of a medical treatise published in 1612, the *Treatise on Hermaphrodites* [*Traité des hermaphrodits*] by a physician from the Norman town of Évreux, Jacques Duval. The author himself admits the text has a powerful erotic charge.

How does the text programme sexual arousal and joy in a reader who is invited mentally to perform the movements described on the stage of proprioception, and to experience them on a cognitive and sensorial level? How does the text appeal to the reader's "kinesic intelligence," promoting the virtual haptics of the act of reading? For Duval taps into the two founding senses of the tradition of anatomical observation, sight and touch, to define a specific form of kinesic experience, establishing a dichotomy between the story being told and the textual effects it provokes. In his role as protagonist, the physician tries to palpate the inside of the hermaphroditic body, without seeing anything, in order to determine its true nature, but in his role as author, he tries to "make [people] touch, as if with the finger and to [make them] see, as if with the eye" the body he describes, through a dynamic and synesthetic exploration.

However, if this text aims to provoke a pluralist perceptual simulation for the reader, it simultaneously problematizes it. The *Traité des hermaphrodits* seems to constitute a real challenge to kinesic intelligence. Following Jean-Marie Goulemot's *Ces Lives qu'on ne lit que d'une main*, a study of pornographic reading in the eighteenth century, I will thus examine the medical text in terms of a "reading position which writing itself imposes" or rather in terms of the reading *positions*, the coenesthetic movements of the reader, which the act of reading makes *possible*—or *impossible*."[5] In fact, the gestures in question concern a being that defies the categories of gender that memory provides, and the text itself is generically hybrid, oscillating between didactic aims and salacious suggestions. These complex or even contradictory movements are akin to the "kinesic opacity" underlined in the introduction to this volume that stimulates the critical consciousness of the sometimes limited mechanisms of cognition and of the ideological prejudices informing it. More broadly, it encourages us to question the role played by the reader's identity—his moral and gendered identity—when employing his kinesic intelligence. Might not the norms of propriety hinder the interior simulation of the described movements, or even suppress it? And might the actions related to the hermaphrodite's "questionable" body not disturb the categories of gender according to which the reader usually views his erotic life, be it real or imagined?

As for how the real reader, and not the inscribed one, reacts and acts in concrete terms, Goulemot's title implies that he is reading with only one hand, moving from mental simulation to practical stimulation. Natural philosophy helps to elucidate the "acting out" specific to erotic literature, since it aims to theorize the physiological conditions of the act of reception by explaining the organic repercussions of a book or an image.

The Eye and the Finger

The main story in Duval's text is the famous case of Marie/Marin le Marcis. Marie wore girls' clothes for twenty-one years before converting to a new gender, at the same time choosing a new name and deciding to renounce his Protestant faith. The person now called Marin le Marcis undertakes administrative steps that allow him to marry. He is handed over to the law. In 1601, he was sentenced to death on the basis of two expert reports, for "the crime of sodomy" ("crime de Sodomie"), "violation of nature" ("viol de Nature"), offense to "public honesty" ("honnesteté publique") and imposture.[6] Jacques Duval, a respected provincial physician, appears on the scene when Marin le Marcis appeals to the court, and forces it to convene a new cohort of experts: six physicians, two surgeons and two obstetricians under oath.[7] Among them, the Rouennais physician stands out when he orchestrates a spectacular recognition scene. He unveils the existence of a retractile penis, which is withdrawn into the body. A masturbation session, administered by science, brings a hermaphrodite into the world. In the wake of Michel Foucault and Stephen Greenblatt, this extraordinary case has attracted the attention of criticism mainly from the perspectives of cultural history and the history of science.[8] Keeping in mind the way literature shapes the presentation of knowledge,

I would like instead to assess the performative impact of the gestures, both physical and rhetorical, which the book presents and which appeal to "the touch of reading."[9] The physician, as we will see, problematizes the relationship between sight and touch, which are usually linked in the anatomical tradition, and he does so in an original manner.

Duval replaces the external examination of Marin le Marcis's body with a "digital" exploration of his (or her) depths.[10] This gesture fits in with the biblical tradition of Doubting Thomas, who is invited to see the holes that the nails of the Cross have left and to put his finger inside them and into Christ's wound (John 20:25)—a scene depicted by Caravaggio. The title of Duval's chapter indicates: "Suitte de la visitation première, et comme l'autheur sonda … avec le doigt" ["Outcome of the first visitation, and how the author probed … with his finger"]. There is a shift from a collective sensual experience ("we felt") to the singularization of perception ("I felt"). The term "author" collapses protagonist and narrator into one and condenses two different temporalities, that of the action (restoring a disputed identity to an outcast) and that of the act of writing. Thus the finger takes on a polysemous value, as an organ of knowledge but also as a writing instrument, a traditional role that it is given in the Judeo-Christian tradition. As Bolens reminds us: the tablets of law entrusted to Moses are written *digito Dei* (Exodus 31:18); Jesus writes with his finger on the ground: *digito scribebat in terra* (John 8:6).

This "multi-purpose" hand has had an emblematic role in the tradition of anatomic illustration ever since the famous self-portrait by Vesalius, a real "signature," as it were, of the *De humani corporis Fabrica*, published in 1543 in Basel by Oporinus (Fig. 7.1).

The anatomist is represented at the threshold of his book, demonstrating the hand muscles. The hand appears both as the object and the subject of knowledge, not only because it carries out the dissection, but also because it writes about and shapes anatomical knowledge, as illustrated by the quill, the inkwell and the text, itself taken from the *Fabrica*, which are located on the little table. We are here witnessing a profound transformation of the value and the aims of dissection: it is now the direct observation of the corpse, the sensorial experience of its flesh—what Jacopo Berengario da Carpi called the *anatomia sensibilis*—that dictates the anatomical text. Notice, as Hélène Cazes does, that Vesalius's look is not directed onto the arm that he is dissecting.[11] It seems instead that he is "looking with his fingertips," in the manner of Jean Riolan the Younger, who informs the reader that he carried out his research "with the help of

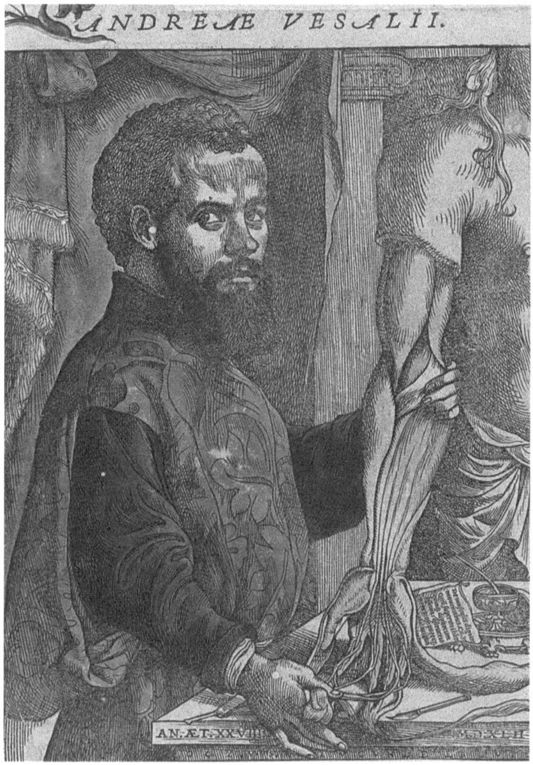

Fig. 7.1 Andreas Vesalius, *De Humani corporis fabrica Libri septem*, Basel, Oporinus, 1543. Universitätsbibliothek Basel, UBH AN I 15

reason and his *ocular hands*."[12] In the eyes of esoteric tradition, as it is articulated in the interpretations of Horapollo's "hieroglyphs," this synaesthetic image reconciles divine omniscience with the human "fabrica." Let us follow Cazes in examining the captions: the eye "comment ilz signifioient Dieu" ["how they signified God"], the hand, "Comment ilz signifioient lhomme qui voluntiers edifie et bastit" ["how they signified man, who readily erects and builds"].[13]

Duval, who refers to his "frequent anatomical dissections," also constantly emphasizes experience and the "authority of the senses" as a source of knowledge.[14] The knowledge of particulars influences the received perception of universals, and case histories reshape the outlines of the category to which they belong.[15] Marin le Marcis thus represents an anomaly in several respects, since "la forme des parties genitales d'iceluy est fort differente de tous les autres filles-hommes ou gynaneres cy dessus mentionnez … " ["the shape of his genital parts is very different from all the other girl-men mentioned above"].[16] The way has been paved by Vesalius, and the physician demonstrates an attitude new to pre-modern Europe: he inverts the traditional relation between theory and empirical observation. Yet in contrast to anatomical tradition, he dissociates eye and finger.

Duval's finger is not the pointing finger that shows and signals things to the sight, but rather the blind finger that touches and discovers a male member, hidden deep within the flesh. The Wittgensteinian dichotomy between *saying* and *showing* is subverted by this finger, which speaks by touching. It even allows Duval to predicate the subject correctly by making it ejaculate (a decisive criterion for determining an individual's gender): the finger mediatizes both the desire for knowledge and the understanding of the object of experimentation. The fundamental and inherent meaning of the finger's touch will continue to be favoured by the great philosophical "tactilist" or "haptocentric" tradition right up to Husserl. Derrida writes on this topic: "In the question of touch …, man is virtually the sole subject, and above all the fingers of his hand."[17]

For Duval, the polarity between the exterior and the interior of the body corresponds to a devaluation of the organ of sight as a passive source of knowledge in favour of what he calls the "force du tact," the active power of touch.[18] This goes against tradition: in the *Quaestiones medico-legales* (1621–51), written by the protophysician of the papal state, Paolo Zacchia, who relates a number of cases of sexual ambiguity, the sense of sight holds a pivotal position as an organ of observation, in accordance with popularly held opinion, dating back to Aristotle and Thomas Aquinas. Touch, by contrast, is considered as the most ordinary and least refined of the senses ("comunissimus") and is accorded little attention.[19]

Duval, however, suggests a new sensory hierarchy that dislodges the legitimate conditions of practice and of medical knowledge, while blurring the generic categorization of his account: it is not so much an *observatio* (although this would not exclude senses other than sight), but it should more rightly be called a *palpatio* or a *tactus intimus*, where the finger, in accordance with its etymology, speaks, or rather makes the body speak. For "doigt" ("finger") is generally derived from the form *deig*—or *deik*—which is related to the verb *dicere*, "to say," "to speak."

This conflict between *seeing* and *feeling* is visible in the dispute that sets Duval against Riolan, an eminent professor of the medical faculty of Paris, who tries to put the little provincial "practicus" in his place with his *Discours sur les hermaphrodits, où il est démontré contre l'opinion commune, qu'il n'y a point de vrays hermaphrodits* [*Discourse on hermaphrodites: Where it is demonstrated, against common opinion, that there are no real hermaphrodites*].[20] He accuses his provincial colleague of imprecision regarding the description of internal organs that have never been anatomized, and with the problematic identification of a penis that remains invisible. According to him, Marin le Marcis is a woman who has an interior tumour, and Duval confuses the discharge of sperm with that of uterine fluids.

The Touch of Reading

For his part, Duval does not content himself with defending fondling as an investigative procedure, and even calls for a "tactile" reading that should not be reduced to language's traditional powers of hypotyposis. He displays the anatomy of the genitals before his readers, as he declares in the first part of his work, in order to "contenter les curieux … en intention de leur *faire toucher quasi du doigt, et veoir comme de l'œil*" ["satisfy the curious … so as to make them touch as if with their finger, and see as if with their eyes"].[21] The author thus defines the mode of action that is specific to his text and aims to programme the reader's sensory experience. He invites us to think about what is at stake in this haptic reading, in this palpation by sight, which invites the reader to prolong the sensory experience of the anatomist.

In French idioms, the eye and the finger have been associated since the fifteenth century: we find "monstrer a l'œil et au doy," "chercher au doy et a l'œil [la plus belle de dame de France]." There is also a legal formula: "monstrer le dit heritege ou maison au doigt et à l'œil." Furetière's dictionary (1690) first records the expression "faire toucher au doigt et à l'œil, montrer au doigt et à l'œil," which means "to show perceptibly to sight and touch." In the dictionary of the Académie (1694), we again find, this time in the abstract sense, "faire connaître au doigt et à l'œil," "faire toucher une vérité au doigt et à l'œil," which is to say "to show it clearly, to prove beyond doubt." However, when the movements of eye and finger are dissociated, they betray foolishness rather than produce real knowledge: in the fifteenth century, we find *se ferir en l'œil son propre doit* (Martin

Le Franc), and in Cotgrave (1611) *se donner du doigt dans l'œil*, to stigmatize the behaviour of the ignorant or foolish.[22] So what role does this conventional mode of expression play in a medical context where the two organs are emblems for understanding with the help of the senses?

The solidarity between eye and finger is mentioned on the one hand regarding the manual expertise of midwives when giving a ruling on the virginity of young women ("Et le tout veu & visité *au doit, & a l'œil*" ["And the whole thing seen and explored by finger and eye"]).[23] On the other hand, it is transposed onto the power of discourse and its effect on the reader, who "visits" the text, which mediates the medical visit of the body. "Visiter" (to examine, to observe with care) also had the meaning of "to read" in sixteenth-century French: one "visits" a letter or letters (Huguet's dictionary), or a book. In Bouvard's work, written in alexandrines, *Description de la maladie, de la mort et de la vie de Madame la Duchesse de Mercoeur, decedée en son Chasteau d'Anet le 6 septembre 1623* [*Description of the illness, the death and the life of Madame the Duchess of Mercoeur who died in her castle in Anet, on the sixth of September 1623*] one can, for instance, read in the dedication: "To Monsieur de Vendosme … since only a physician can see clearly concerning the knowledge of illnesses, their causes, events and remedies …, that is why *je le vous fais voir à l'œil et toucher au doigt par ceste description*" (a literal translation of this phrase would be: "I will make you see it with the eye and touch it with the finger with the help of this description.")[24] Poetic power guarantees continuity from the physician's experience to that of the reader. In Duval, the double modalization—*quasi du doigt, comme de l'œil*—points to the gap that separates the experience of the real body from that of the imagined body, but also to the similarity of their proprioceptive effects. Moreover, the co-text revives the set phrase by reliteralizing it: the most striking experience of the work, Duval's digital exploration—the blind reading with his finger—is to be extended in the reading experience of the book, which allows the reader to perform again mentally the physical realities (gestures, fondling, contact) presented in the account. At the same time that Duval introduces his finger into the hermaphrodite, the reader follows the successions of signs on the page with his finger and, following the example of the Apostle Thomas, begins to believe. The optical act of reading, assisted by the hand, is supposed to lead to a haptic sensation. The reader literally has to put his finger in his eye, to awaken the touch of the eye, which becomes a finger, in order to palpate in his turn the ambiguous body of Marin le Marcis.[25] In short the text is, paradoxically, destined to make the reader see (in order to enable him to touch) that which has remained invisible to the protagonist, or rather to ***make the reader see that which the protagonist could not see.*** The kinesic intelligence thus mobilizes the perceptual means rejected at the level of the story in order to demonstrate their uselessness more fully.

A Problematic Discovery

And yet this fondling gesture, which brings to light a hermaphrodite, proves doubly problematic when envisaged from within the paradigm of anagnorisis, described by Terence Cave in *Recognitions*.[26] Consequently, the manner in which the reader's kinesic knowledge is mobilized becomes more complex.

Firstly, Duval's investigative gesture constitutes a paradox. It restores a masculine role to Marin le Marcis by means of a procedure that assigns him a traditionally feminine role. According to Caspar Bauhin, who is seeking criteria to assign a gender to a hermaphrodite: "Nam si vulva … pervia sit, ut virile membrum admittere possit … planè foeminae judicantur" ["If the vulva can be penetrated, so that the male organ can enter …, they can fully be considered as women."][27] The finger which is thrust into Marin le Marcis's lower abdomen thus reveals his masculinity even as it reaffirms her femininity. How is this gender trouble, to borrow a term from Judith Butler, likely to affect the kinesic understanding of the reader? And to what extent is kinesic intelligence gendered when the reader is confronted with such sexual scenarios?

Secondly, Duval's gesture goes against the norms of decency and cannot be spoken of without precautions, even if, according to Foucault, Duval's examination offers "the very first rudiments of a clinical approach to sexuality" where each thing is called by its name.[28] Indeed, the description of the hermaphrodite's ejaculation, brought about by a second fondling, is shrouded in a multiplicity of subordinate clauses. This gesture, which is offered to the reader's simulation, is muffled under layers of syntax and constrained by psychological and social taboos.

> Et voyant le refus d'y toucher, outre ce que je feus curieux lors, de m'attribuer plus exacte cognoissance d'une chose tant rare, et dont je n'avois memoire qu'aucun autheur eust fait mention, pour m'appuyant d'avantage en cette sentence, y demeurer ferme, ou du tout m'en departant adherer à l'opinion de ceux qui jugeoient n'y avoir rien de viril audict suject, j'y remis le doigt

pour la seconde fois, en laquelle ayant trouvé laditte partie tellement disposee, qu'aucun doutte ne m'en pouvoit rester, jusques à avoir veu ledit Marin stimulé qu'il fut par frequente attrectation, espandre semence genitale blanche, espesse, et mediocrement fluide, telle en fin que Aristote qui la constituë seul principe seminal, la descrit au commencement du quatriesme *De generatione animalum* Non aqueuse en qualité tant fluide ny sereuse comme la femme a accoustumé render.[29]

[And regarding the refusal to touch it, beyond the fact that I was curious to attribute to myself a more exact knowledge of a thing so rare, and which I had no memory of another author mentioning, for better positioning myself in this judgment, to stay firm in it, or in altogether departing from it to adhere to the opinion of those who judged that there was nothing of the male in the subject, I re-inserted my finger for the second time, this time having found the said part disposed, such that no doubt could remain with me, to the point of having seen the said Marin stimulated as he was by repeated touching, spill generative seed that was white, viscous, and indifferently liquid, just as Aristotle, for whom it constitutes the sole seminal source, described at the beginning of the fourth book of *De generatione animalum*. Neither aqueous in quality of fluid, nor serous, such as that a woman is accustomed to make.]

Like a cat on a hot tin roof, Duval skids over the decisive fact that establishes the hermaphrodite's identity. He frames Marin le Marcis's stimulation (which is carefully formulated in the passive form "stimulé qu'il fut …") by affirming the purity of his intentions and by referring to the authority of Aristotle. The accompanying discourse justifying the intrepid exploration is nearly as long as the description itself: Duval relates his inner struggle, taking refuge behind Aristotle, and then recalls his request "vers la compagnie, qu'elle n'attribuast à indiscretion, ou cogitation lascive, si je mettois le doigt dedans la partie" ["of the company, that it not be attributed to indiscretion, or to lascivious thoughts, if I inserted my finger into those parts"].[30] This denial of any emotional involvement applies both to the teratoscopy and to the discourse, as a note to the reader signals:

…si j'uses [*sic*] de propos qui paroissent lascifs, ou ressentent quelque gayeté, dont puissent tant soit peu estre offencez les oreilles … ce que j'en faicts, n'est pour aucune affection lascive qui soit en moy.[31]

[…if I had dealings that appear lascivious, or express some frivolousness which could even slightly offend the ears … what I did with them was not for any lascivious sensation in myself.]

The purity that guides the practitioner's gestures thus corresponds to that of the rhetorical "gestures"—to take up Quintilian's definition for figures of speech—which abound in Duval's text.[32] For instance, it is at the moment of the sexual act that the voracity of the "matrix" (that is, the uterus) manifests itself most clearly, with the lascivity of an amorous mouth, the frisky grace of an insect, the undulation of a fish:

> Cette bouche s'ouvre aisément, librement et voluptueusement, quand il est question de recevoir le sperme viril, dont elle est friande et avide merveilleusement. Occasion pour laquelle l'homme la sent au coït voltigeant comme un papillon ou mouvant comme une tanche, pour lui venir par intervalles baiser et sucer l'extrémité du balanus, prétendant avoir son baume naturel.[33]
>
> [This mouth opens easily, freely and voluptuously, when it is a question of receiving the male seed, for which it is wonderfully greedy and eager. An instance in which the man feels a coupling that is fluttering like a butterfly or moving like a tench, by intervals kissing and sucking the extremity of the glans, desiring to have his natural balm.]

The text adopts the perspective of a man who "feels," in an infra-visual manner, the motion and suction of the matrix. The mouth of the butterfly or tench combines synecdoche with comparison and stresses the tension between contradictory registers: bucolic and amorous on the one hand, obscene, aquatic and viscous on the other. The animal and human realms overlap to raise the matrix from its status of organ to that of a being endowed with an autonomous vitality all of its own.

Reading as Simulation: Acting Out

The reader thus faces a medical text which constantly offers narrativized sexual actions, favourable to stimulation and imaginary simulation. Yet the experience that Duval offers is full of ambiguity. In a contradictory double movement, the physician wants to prove his intentions innocent, while at the same time acknowledging that any text addressing sexual matters will invariably titillate the reader.

> La puissante nature [...] a, par je ne sçay quel instinct, concedé une tant voluptueuse titillation et libidineuse amorce, lors que par la nomination, ou seule signification [des parties sexuelles], l'esprit est attiré à s'y encliner, que quand j'userois de lettres Hierogliphiques empruntees des Egyptiens, ou

seulement de signes expressifs repetés de l'Anglois Taumaste, pour les designer, sans autrement les nommer: encores ne pourrois-je rescinder cette naïfve gayeté dont nature a voulu decorer et orner leur commemoration.[34]

[Powerful Nature [...] has, by I know not what instinct, lent by association a voluptuous titillation and libidinous bait [to sexual parts], a bait that the spirit seizes upon at the naming or mere signification [of sexual parts], in such a way that if I were to use hieroglyphs borrowed from the Egyptians, or just the expressive repeating symbols of the Englishman Taumaste, to designate [sexual parts], without otherwise naming them: I still could not counteract this native lightness with which nature wished to garland and embellish their commemoration.]

The *intentio operis*—what the text is saying, irrespective of its author's intentions—exonerates the *intentio auctoris*. The narrator does not want to be associated with the reader's fantasies, although he caters to them with perfect ambiguity.

Reading is thus not an activity purely of the mind, which frees one from one's corporeal reality. Duval himself insists on the connection between intellectual activities and the senses. He quotes Aristotle, who acknowledges "que la pensee et intellect a grande connexité avec le sentiment ... Et pour le faire court il veut qu'il n'y ait rien en l'entendement qui n'ait esté premierement au sens" ["that thought and the intellect are closely connected to feeling [...] And in short he claims that there is nothing in the understanding that was not already first in the senses"].[35] Contemporary libertine texts often point to their own carnal power in light of precisely this connection. "By a new custom/Your prose—excuse my French—fucks us through the eyes": thus concludes the dedicatory madrigal from the *École des filles* in the middle of the seventeenth century.[36]

This idea is nothing new. It joins a priapic tradition in which *The Hermaphroditus* of Panormita (Antonio Beccadelli)—a heretical collection of epigrams modelled on Martial and the Priapeia—plays a tragic role, given that it was one of the first texts to be burned on grounds of obscenity, at the injunction of Pope Eugene IV in 1431.

In the *Hermaphroditus* the genitals become attributes of the book itself: "Cunnus et est nostro, simul est et mentula, libro" ["This book is at once a prick and a cunt"] (Her. 1.3.3).[37] Epigram 37 is addressed to the book itself, "so that it may go to the brothel of Florence." The first verse, "i, fuge," refers to the Ovidian topos of *Vade, liber*, "Go, my book," and the Horatian *Fuge*, in which the Latin poet addresses the book (liber) as a child (liber), charged with revealing to the readers at the end of the epistle that it is he, Horace. But unlike the Horatian book, which mediates between the poet and his public, Panormita's book has its own autonomous and ebullient life:

> On your vulva and on your member, because you have both,
> Galla, without blushing, will place her hand.
> [...]
> At last, a troop of all the whores in this noble city
> Will surround you, delighted at your arrival.
> You can tell them filthy little nothings and make them happen,
> No refusal will bring a blush to your face.
> There, just as you have wished and wanted for so long,
> You will fuck and be fucked as you desire, my book.
> (Quantum vis futues et futuere, liber).[38]

Far from reconciling itself to choosing one of two sexes as ordained by both canon and civil law, the book will "draw double pleasure" from its expedition.

The act of reading resembles a sexual experience that mobilizes, through synaesthesia, the entire sensory range. *To let oneself be fucked through the eyes* means to surrender to a *total* embrace that transcends the too-narrow confines of a traditional anthropology fixated on visual fantasy. Therefore, the sentences not only *imprint* themselves onto the brain or "*paint* onto the imagination, as strongly as Michelangelo could have done it on canvas, the dirty and brutal action which produces the pregnancy of [a] girl."[39] Here, the sentences are making love to the reader, even if it means driving him to quite concrete sexual actions, a phenomenon that the ancient theory of sympathy partly clarifies. The seventh book of the *Problemata*, a famous text attributed to Aristotle, which was edited and translated numerous times during the Renaissance, is devoted to the effects of *sympatheia*. Its author emphasizes the spontaneous and involuntary imitation of activities perceived by the senses:

> Why do men generally themselves yawn when they see others yawn? Is it because, if they are reminded of it when they feel a desire to perform any function, they then put it into execution, particularly where the desire is easily stirred, for example, that of passing urine? ... Or does this not always occur, but only when the body happens to feel a desire and is in such a condition that its moisture becomes heated? For then it is recollection which

gives the impulse, as also in sexual desire and hunger; for it is that which causes recollection to exist that provides the stimulus towards the object [pathos] in our imagination.[40]

Reconfiguring the sensory data (among which could be counted the act of reading linguistic signs on a page), the imagination produces a representation that awakens the recollection of a similar real-life experience, lodged in the reservoir of memory. This recollection "gives the [physical] impulse" and prompts the nerves to imitate "the object [pathos] in our imagination." The sexual act and the act of feeding obey the same impulsive behaviour, where the rational being is subjected to a blind physiological drive, "the savage law of sympathy."[41] Girolamo Fracastoro picks up on this analogy between different domains of instinctive life in his *De sympathia et antipathia rerum*.[42] His theory allows us to understand the phenomena of kinesic empathy at the level of concrete action (as opposed to that of mental simulation).

The sensual effectiveness of a text is undoubtedly a function of the power of its style (in the poetic and rhetorical sense). It certainly also depends on historically determined conceptualizations of the body, which inform the narration (for the author) and the mental simulation that it brings about (for the reader). A specific knowledge of the body is mobilized in order to tell stories, but also to devour them.

By making his main subject a spectacular *observatio*, accompanied by a series of other hermaphrodite "stories" taken from his own direct experience, Duval becomes part of a fashionable new literary genre that flourishes from the second part of the sixteenth century onwards, namely that of *Historiae* and *Observationes*. This printing boom reflects the new cognitive value conferred on the recording of personal experience and the success of a sensory epistemology in the field of medicine and anatomy, whose emblems are the finger (or the hand) and the eye. This change has repercussions for the representation of the act of reading, which has to mobilize the different senses of the recipient beyond the mere instrument of sight, the most intellectual of the senses. At the same time, the kinesic experience offered by Duval's text calls for some complicated, variegated and disconcerting mental gymnastics. First, because it offers role-plays to the reader, where the borders of gender are uncertain and can conflict with the manner in which he mobilizes his own gendered identity in the act of kinesic interpretation. Confronted with a conventional erotic scenario, the reader is free to try on a role belonging specifically to the other sex, to replay it internally in order to "perform gender," to use Judith Butler's terminology.[43] Yet given the strange relationship that develops between Duval and the hermaphrodite, the reader's own perception of the differences between the sexes is troubled, as is the possibility of labelling a movement as either definitely feminine or masculine.

Second, kinesic intelligence is further challenged because the study of the hermaphrodite, that mixed being, shapes the ambiguous genre of the narrative, which acknowledges its power of arousal while at the same time flaunting its didactic purity. How do the norms of propriety hinder the free internal movement of the reader? The model of kinesic stimulation is mobilized, yet a certain methodological prudence seems required: the aim is not to universalize the process of reading or to erase the reader's historicity. By reconciling the theoretical models of cognitive anthropology and a historical approach to the experience of reading, it may become possible to describe two phenomena: on the one hand, the remarkable enduring power of the erotic texts of the past, including Duval's text.[44] For their power to act upon the senses and the mind of the modern reader seems unimpaired—a longevity that Jean-Marie Goulemot calls the "transhistoricity of the obscene" and which Joseph Bédier deplores as the "unbelievable monotony of human obscenity."[45] On the other hand, there is the specificity of the act of reading in the seventeenth century, conditioned by representations and cultural norms belonging to the epistemology and the morals of its time. The actual reception of Duval's text—it was seized by a ruling of parliament on 4 April 1612 and sales were suspended—and the figure of the narratee that it constructs clearly illustrate this second phenomenon.

Yet nothing allows us to measure the individual reader's mimetic fidelity with regard to the movements described in the text: is not everyone, in their own manner, likely to reproduce, or simulate internally, *less* than what is being said (for reasons of decency or self-censorship) or *more*, when the *fantasia*, the creative power that can freely reconstruct the species perceived by the senses and actively create new forms, prevails over the imagination, which contents itself with receiving and reproducing the data provided by the senses? How, then, should we parse phantasmatic activity and kinesic intelligence? Considering this particular form of intelligence within a Renaissance context means taking into account the creative, uncontrollable and irrational power accorded to the *fantasia*. Might not that faculty be able to prolong, amplify or even trigger movements that are not necessarily present in the text itself?

Notes

1. Guillemette Bolens, *Le Style des gestes. Corporéité et kinésie dans le récit littéraire* (Paris: Éditions BHMS, 2010), 10. Bolens cites Jean Decety and Julie Grèzes, "The Power of Simulation: Imagining One's Own and Other's Behavior," *Brain Research* 1079 (2006): 4–14.
2. François Vanoosthuyse, "Littérature et Kinésie," *Critique, "Du style!"* 752–3 (January–February 2010): 160. For a bibliography on the subject, see also Bolens, *Le Style des gestes*, 11.
3. In noting that "peut-être la notion de corporéité devrait-elle recouvrir davantage de champs que ce que Guillemette Bolens envisage," ["perhaps the notion of corporeality should be thought to extend over more extensive territory than Guillemette Bolens envisages], Vanoosthuyse gives first place to erotic literature; "Littérature et kinésie," 167.
4. Vanoosthuyse, "Littérature et Kinésie."
5. Jean-Marie Goulemot, *Ces livres qu'on ne lit que d'une main. Lecture et lecteurs de livres pornographiques au xviiie siècle* (Paris: Alinéa, 1991), 7.
6. Jacques Duval, *Des hermaphrodits, accouchemens de femmes, et traitement qui est requis pour les relever en santé* (Rouen: David Geuffroy, 1612), 397. The only modern republication is *Traité des hermaphrodits, parties génitales, accouchemens des femmes, etc.*, (Paris: Liseux, 1880). The trial began on 7 January and ended on 7 June 1601.
7. Note the order: the first visit was by two surgeons, the second by a doctor, an apothecary and two surgeons; Duval, *Traité des hermaphrodits*, 400.
8. Michel Foucault, *Les Anormaux. Cours au Collège de France. 1974–1975* (Paris: Seuil-Gallimard, 1999), 62–6. Stephen Greenblatt, "Fiction and Friction," in *Reconstructing Individualism. Autonomy, Individuality, and the Self in Western Thought*, ed. T. C. Heller, M. Sosna, D. E. Wellberry (Stanford: Stanford University Press, 1986), 30–52.
9. The other studies devoted to Duval's treatise are cited in this analysis, with the exception of the excellent study of discursive forms and the question of linguistic taboos by Joseph Harris, "La force du tact': Representing the Taboo Body in Jacques Duval's *Traité des Hermaphrodits* (1612)," *French Studies* 72, no. 3 (2003): 311–22; concerning Duval's discursive skill, Kathleen P. Long, *Hermaphrodites in Renaissance Europe* (Hampshire, England/Burlington, USA: Ashgate, 2006), 86–90.
10. The scene of the "visitation" extends, with consummate use of suspense, over three chapters (66–8).
11. Hélène Cazes, *L'Œil et la main, Anatomies 16–18, 14 décembre 2012*, accessed March 28, 2016, https://oeiletmain.files.wordpress.com/2012/10/pistes-et-documents.pdf.

12. Jean Riolan, *Manuel anatomique et pathologique, ou abregé de toute l'anatomie* (Lyon: Antoine Laurens, 1672), "Advertissement au Lecteur et Auditeur." See Rafael Mandressi, "Le corps des savants. Science, histoire, performance," *Communications* 92, no. 1 (2013): 52.
13. Horapollo, *De la signification des notes hiéroglyphiques des Aegyptiens,... nouvellement traduict de grec en francoys et imprimé avec les figures chacun chapitre*, trans. J. Martin. Paris, J. Kerver, 1543, f. n iij. et n.p.
14. Duval, *Traité des Hermaphrodits*, 51; 301 (on the dissection of hares). On 425–6 he responds to those who reproach him with the examples of the "Anatomistes" (Sylvius, Bauhin, Colomb) who have carried out "la dissection des parties interieures des Hermaphrodits" ["the dissection of the inner parts of hermaphrodites"].
15. On this development, see Gianna Pomata, "Sharing Cases: the *Observationes* in Early Modern Medicine," *Early Science and Medicine* 15 (2010): 232; Duval, *Traité des hermaphrodits*, 302: "Puis que nous avons remarqué par les histoires qu'il s'engendre des Hermaphrodits" ["Since we have observed from case histories that hermaphrodites are engendered"].
16. *Ibid.*, 383. In this particular form, the male member has the ability to retract into and protrude from the interior of the body.
17. Jacques Derrida, *Le Toucher, Jean-Luc Nancy* (Paris: Galilée, 2000), 192. My translation.
18. Duval, *Traité des hermaphrodits,* 409.
19. Alessandro Pastore, "Sens et expérience dans les *Quaestiones* de Paolo Zacchia," forthcoming in *Hermes medicus. Discours et actions de l'herméneutique médicale (xve-xviie)*, ed. A. Carlino (Amsterdam-New York: Rodopi).
20. (Paris, Pierre Ramier, 1614).
21. Duval, *Traité des hermaphrodits*, 3.
22. Gilles Roques, "L'œil dans les locutions et expressions françaises," *Cahier des Annales de Normandie. Mélanges René Lepelley* 26 (1995): 380–81, accessed 30 August 2014, http://www.persee.fr/web/revues/home/prescript/article/annor_0570-1600_1995_hos_26_1_2283
23. Laurent Joubert, *Erreurs Populaires* (Bordeaux: Simon Millanges, 1578), 467–8.
24. "Pource qu'il n'y a que le Medecin seul qui voye clair en la cognoissance des maladies, de leurs causes, evenements et remedes [...]" (Paris, Jean Libert, 1624), aiv^{r}.
25. For the finger in the eye in another context, see "Le corps et la toile, ou le corps du peintre dans l'art contemporain (Pollock, Johns, Lichtenstein, Art corporel)," in *Les Figures du corps dans la littérature et la peinture anglaises et américaines,* ed. B. Brugière (Paris: Publications de la Sorbonne, 1991), 326. For the dichotomy between seeing and touching, see also Maurice Merleau-Ponty, *Le Visible et l'invisible* (Paris: Gallimard, 1964).

26. Terence Cave, *Recognitions. A Study in Poetics* (Oxford: Clarendon Press, 1988).
27. Caspar Bauhin, *De Hermaphroditorum monstrorumque partuum natura* (Oppenheim: Galler, De Bry, 1614), cited by Long, *Hermaphrodites in Renaissance Europe*, 57.
28. Foucault, *Les Anormaux*, 63.
29. Duval, *Traité des hermaphrodits*, chap. 68: "Suitte de la visitation premiere et comme l'hauteur [sic] sonda les parties naturelles dudit Marin le Marcis avec le doigt, en quoy faisant il trouva son membre viril et de sa situation," ["The continuation of the first examination and how the author investigated the natural parts of the said Marin le Marcis with his finger, by doing which he found his virile member and its location"], 404–5.
30. "Et ne fus reprimé d'aucune honte, memoratif de la sentence d'Aristote sur la fin du premier livre des parties des animaux et de leurs causes. Où il blasme les Philosophes, qui ont laissé arriere la consideration de quelques animaux, et des parties d'iceux, pour leur sembler deshonnestes à l'attouchement, et vergongneuses à l'exposition," ["And I was touched by no shame, since I remembered Aristotle's declaration at the end of the first book of the parts of the animals and their causes, where he condemns philosophers who have not considered some animals and their parts on account of their appearing unseemly to touch, and shameful to discuss."]; Duval, 402–3.
31. Duval, "Advertissement au Lecteur."
32. According to Quintilien, the word "figure … s'applique à des attitudes et, pourrait-on dire, à des gestes [du langage]," *Institution oratoire,* tome v, books VIII et IX, ed. and trans. J. Cousin (Paris: Les Belles Lettres, 1978), 159.
33. Duval, *Des hermaphrodits*, chap. 15: "Du corps de la matrice, de son orifice, sa louange, et des signes de conception" ["On the body of the uterus, its orifice, its praise, and of signs of conception"], 107.
34. Duval, "Advertissement au Lecteur."
35. Duval, 409.
36. Extract cited by Harris, "'La force du tact'": 314. On *L'École des filles*, probably written by Claude le Petit, see Michel Jeanneret, *Eros rebelle. Littérature et dissidence à l'ère classique* (Paris: Seuil, 2003), 217–18, and more generally chapter 8, "Livres aphrodisiaques."
37. *Antonio Beccadelli, Hermaphroditus*, ed. and trans. E. O'Connor (Lenham, Maryland: Lexington Books, 2001 [1925]), 19.
38. *L'Hermaphrodite de Panormita (xvie siècle), traduit pour la première fois avec le texte latin et un choix de notes de Forberg* (Paris: Isidore Liseux, 1892), 2: 119.
39. Pierre Bayle, *Dictionnaire historique et critique*, 11th ed. (Paris: Beuchot, 1820), 657.

40. Aristotle, *Problemata*, trans. E. S. Forster (Oxford: Clarendon Press, 1927), vii, 1–2, 886a, 24–35, accessed 28 March 2016, https://archive.org/stream/workstranslatedi07arisuoft/workstranslatedi07arisuoft_djvu.txt. I have corrected the last sentence, which is erroneous ("towards the condition observed in another person"). For a commentary on this passage see Roberto Poma, *Magie et guérison. La rationalité de la médecine magique (xvie–xviie siècles)* (Paris: Orizons, 2009), 229–32.
41. Aristotle, 232.
42. Girolamo Fracastor, *Liber I de sympathia et antiphatia rerum, de contagione et contagiosis morbis, et eorum curatione libri tres* (Lyon: Guillaume Gazel, 1550), "De aliis quibusdam consensibus phantasiae," 199. The parallel between the two texts is proposed by Giulio Guastavini, a collaborator with Casaubon, in his *Commentarii in priores decem Aristotelis Problematum sectiones* (Lyon: Horace Cardon, 1608), 273.
43. Judith Butler, *Gender Trouble: Feminism and the Subversion of Identity* (London: Routledge, 1990); see the last chapter in particular.
44. Alain Berthoz, in his preface to Bolens's *Le Style des gestes*, stresses the eclecticism of the examples she analyses, but defends them as necessary in order to show the universality of "corporéité et de la kinésie dans le récit littéraire" ["corporeity and kinesis in literary narrative"]; Bolens, *Le Style des gestes*, xii. It is true that the author is concerned with showing the applicability of an ahistorical cognitive model. On the other hand, Daniel Punday insists on the historical character of his perspective in his important study *Narrative Bodies: Toward a Corporeal Narratology* (New York-Basingstoke, Hampshire: Macmillan, 2003). Punday demonstrates the relationship between narrativization, reading and the conception of the body, and how textual accounts reflect the epistemological conditions of specific historic moments; *Narrative Bodies*, 11.
45. Goulemot, *Ces livres qu'on ne lit que d'une main*, 9; Joseph Bédier, *Les Fabliaux: études de littérature populaire et d'histoire littéraire du Moyen Âge* (Paris: E. Bouillon, 1893), 358.

Bibliography

Aristotle. *Problemata*. Translated by E. S. Forster. Oxford: Clarendon Press, 1927

Bauhin, Caspar. *De Hermaphroditorum Monstrorumque Partuum Natura*. Oppenheim: Galler for De Bry, 1614.

Bayle, Pierre. *Dictionnaire historique et critique*. 11th ed. Paris: Beuchot, 1820.

Beccadelli, Antonio. *L'Hermaphrodite de Panormita (xvie siècle), traduit pour la première fois avec le texte latin et un choix de notes de Forberg*. Paris: Isidore Liseux, 1892.

———. *Hermaphroditus*. Edited and Translated by E. O'Connor. 1925; repr. Lenham, Maryland: Lexington Books, 2001.

Bédier, Joseph. *Les Fabliaux: études de littérature populaire et d'histoire littéraire du Moyen Âge*. Paris: E. Bouillon, 1893.

Bolens, Guillemette. *Le Style des gestes. Corporéité et kinésie dans le récit littéraire.* Paris: Éditions BHMS, 2010.

Bouvard, Charles. *Description de la maladie, de la mort et de la vie de Mme la duchesse de Mercoeur, décédée en son château d'Anet, le 6 septembre 1623.* Paris: J. Sibert, 1624.

Brancher, Dominique. *Equivoques de la pudeur. Fabrique d'une passion à la Renaissance*. Geneva: Droz, 2015.

Brugière, B. *Les Figures du corps: dans la littérature et la peinture anglaises et américaines*. Paris: Publications de la Sorbonne, 1991.

Butler, Judith. *Gender Trouble: Feminism and the Subversion of Identity*. London: Routledge, 1990.

Cave, Terence. *Recognitions. A Study in Poetics.* Oxford: Clarendon Press, 1988.

Cazes, Hélène. *L'Œil et la main, Anatomies 16–18, 14 décembre* 2012. Accessed 28 March 2016. https://oeiletmain.files.wordpress.com/2012/10/pistes-et-documents.pdf

Decety, Jean, and Julie Grèzes. The Power of Simulation: Imagining One's Own and Other's Behavior. *Brain Research* 1079 (2006): 4–14.

Derrida, Jacques. *Le Toucher, Jean-Luc Nancy*. Paris: Galilée, 2000.

Duval, Jacques. *Des hermaphrodits, accouchemens de femmes, et traitement qui est requis pour les relever en santé.* Rouen: David Geuffroy, 1612.

———. *Traité des hermaphrodits, parties génitales, accouchemens des femmes*, etc. Paris: Liseux, 1880.

Foucault, Michel. *Les Anormaux. Cours au Collège de France. 1974–1975.* Paris: Seuil-Gallimard, 1999.

Fracastor, Jérôme. *Liber I de sympathia et antiphatia rerum, de contagione et contagiosis morbis, et eorum curatione libri tres.* Lyon: Guillaume Gazel, 1550.

Goulemot, Jean-Marie. *Ces livres qu'on ne lit que d'une main. Lecture et lecteurs de livres pornographiques au xviiie siècle.* Paris: Alinéa, 1991.

Greenblatt, Stephen. Fiction and Friction. In *Reconstructing Individualism. Autonomy, Individuality, and the Self in Western Thought.* Edited by T. C. Heller, M. Sosna, and D. E. Wellberry. Stanford: Stanford University Press, 1986.

Grèzes, Julie, and Jean Decety. The Power of Simulation: Imagining One's Own and Other's Behavior. *Brain Research* 1079 (2006): 4–14.

Horapollo. *De la signification des notes hiéroglyphiques des Aegyptiens,... nouvellement traduict de grec en francoys et imprimé avec les figures chacun chapitre.* Translated by J. Martin. Paris: J. Kerver, 1543

Jeanneret, Michel. *Eros rebelle. Littérature et dissidence à l'ère classique*. Paris: Seuil, 2003.

Joubert, Laurent. *Erreurs Populaires.* Bordeaux: Simon Millanges, 1578.

Long, Kathleen P. *Hermaphrodits in Renaissance Europe.* Farnham: Ashgate, 2006.

Mandressi, Rafael. Le corps des savants: Science, histoire, performance. *Communications* 92, no. 1 (2013): 51–65.

Merleau-Ponty, Maurice. *Le Visible et l'invisible.* Paris: Gallimard, 1993.

Pastore, Alessandro. Sens et expérience dans les *Quaestiones* de Paolo Zacchia. In *Hermes medicus. Discours et actions de l'herméneutique médicale (xve–xviie)*, edited by Andrea Carlino. Amsterdam: Rodopi, 2018.

Poma, Roberto. *Magie et guérison. La rationalité de la médecine magique (xvie–xviie siècles).* Paris: Orizons, 2009.

Pomata, Gianna. Sharing Cases: The *Observationes* in Early Modern Medicine. *Early Science and Medicine* 15 (2010): 193–236.

Prévot, J., T. Bedouelle, and E. Wolff (eds.). *Libertins du xviie siècle.* Paris: Gallimard, 1998.

Punday, Daniel. *Narrative Bodies: Toward A Corporeal Narratology.* New York: Macmillan, 2003.

Riolan, Jean. *Manuel anatomique et pathologique, ou abregé de toute l'anatomie.* Lyon: Antoine Laurens, 1672.

Roques, Gilles. L'œil dans les locutions et expressions françaises. *Cahier des Annales de Normandie. Mélanges René Lepelley* 26 (1995): 375–384. Accessed 30 August 2014. http://www.persee.fr/web/revues/home/prescript/article/annor_0570-1600_1995_hos_26_1_2283

Vanoosthuyse, François. Littérature et Kinésie. *Critique, "Du style!"* 752–753 (January–February, 2010): 158–169.

CHAPTER 8

Exchanging Hands in *Titus Andronicus*

Laura Seymour

To Touch and to Know

In one of the most arresting moments in *Titus Andronicus* (first performed 1594), Titus asks Aaron to help him cut off his hand so that he can exchange it for his sons' lives. Titus' words at this point, "Lend me thy hand, and I will give thee mine" (3.1.187), play on the more usual idea of "lending" or "giving" someone one's hand as a figurative term for a handshake whilst also emphasizing that Titus' hand will literally be given as an object of exchange. On one reading, Titus' words simply constitute a dark joke: Titus is mimicking a handshake with a severed hand, and by offhandedly using the casual phrase "lend me thy hand" he is commenting ironically on what is actually happening: rather than a handshake between friends, Aaron is lending his hand to chop off Titus'. Titus continues this dark joke later when he instructs Aaron to "give his majesty my hand" (3.1.194). Rather than proffering his living hand for Saturninus to shake, Titus is sending him his severed hand as a bargaining chip.

Titus and Aaron's handshake fails to live up to the ideals associated with handshakes at the time. In *Titus Andronicus*, Shakespeare dramatizes the consequences of this. Early modern handclasps were associated with

L. Seymour (✉)
Bath Spa University, Bath, UK

K. Banks, T. Chesters (eds.), *Movement in Renaissance Literature*, Cognitive Studies in Literature and Performance,
https://doi.org/10.1007/978-3-319-69200-5_8

honesty, friendship and firm promises, and the reason for this was largely due to the fact that they enabled two people to feel each other's skin. Fundamental to these effects of the handshake was the assumption that clasping each other's hands allowed two people to use touch to get to know each other's hearts and minds. Early modern writers described the handclasp's ability to lay open a person's soul and make it accessible through the touch of living, feeling skin on living, feeling skin. The severed hand that Titus offers Aaron, however, is mere inert matter; it cannot feel or move as a living hand can, and so it cannot truly enable Titus to know Aaron, who tricks him. Titus' severed "handshake" is more than just a throwaway joke: it marks a tragic subversion of friendship, trust, social norms, and Titus' place in society.

Handshakes have been important in our everyday lives since at least the early modern era; Titus' handshake is shocking not just because it is gory but also because it subverts an ordinary, yet crucial aspect of social life. Renaissance texts demonstrate that touching another person's skin was vital for making bargains, marrying and making friends with, and generally getting to know, influence, and be influenced by, that person. In his *History of the World* (1614), for instance, Walter Raleigh shows that the naked hand is the precondition for a "naked" (sincere) bargain,

> When the Earle of *Caesarea* saw that the *Caliph* gaue his hand, neither willingly nor bare, hee told him roundly thus much in effect. SIR, *Truth* needs no holes to hide it selfe; Princes, that will hold couenant, must deale openly, nakedly, and sincerely; Giue vs therefore your bare hand, if you meane that we shall trust you, for we will make no bargaines with your Gloue.[1]

Raleigh plays upon the connotations of the word "naked," which meant not only unclothed, but also sincere and undisguised. Minds are laid open in hands, and the touch and movement of two hands, it seems here, is what enables two minds to interact. The idea that only a person's "naked" skin could enable genuine contact with their mind has persisted through to the present day. In a work on gesture first published in 1807, *Practical Illustrations of Rhetorical Gesture and Action*, the actor Henry Siddons wrote that it had long been thought rude to shake hands with one's gloves on, as the covered hand is entangled with discourses of (dis)honesty, "Persons to this day apologise when they shake hands with their gloves on, and sometimes conclude with this elegant witticism: 'Excuse my glove, perhaps it is the more honest skin of the two.'"[2] In the present day, according to *Etiquette for Dummies*, unless absolutely necessary, gloves must always be removed before shaking hands with someone.[3]

These three examples from across history, one from Shakespeare's time, one from today and one from in between the two, show how grasping the other's hand has been important for cognition across the centuries. Cognitive theories of kinesis remind us (as many early modern texts do too), that a handclasp is not just about touch: it is also about motion. This chapter argues that, during a handshake, movement and (as Raleigh and Siddons emphasize) touch engage the mind with the body according to the principle (to use a formulation in the style of Lakoff and Johnson) TO GRASP is TO KNOW. By grasping the other's hand, we come to know them, to influence them and to let them influence us. Early modern writers saw the ideal handshake as involving a range of embodied ideas of exchange all in play at once: exchange of thoughts, promises, hearts, friendship and love. Cognitive theorists to be discussed below suggest that our bodies do not just provide a visual representation of these psychological exchanges after they have happened; rather, our bodies are where these cognitive acts and experiences actually take place. We do not shake hands to represent a union of minds; our handshake itself is what unifies our minds. Ideally, when we shake hands, then, our skin is not just inert matter—it is our place in society, our ability to "give" ourselves to others and our ability to touch others' minds as well as be touched by theirs.

The idea of kinesic intelligence has been articulated by Guillemette Bolens, who in her *The Style of Gestures* argues that we understand others through their movements (as well as other bodily phenomena such as blushing). We gain this knowledge, she argues, through repeated bodily experiences including engagements with others—watching their bodies and responding with our own, for instance by mimicking their actions to understand them ourselves, kinesic learning—and store our findings in our kinaesthetic memory. She also shows how authors use our ability to understand others, through our own kinesic intelligence and kinaesthetic memories, to understand literary characters.[4] Thus, when we read that a character blushes or springs into the air we know instantly that they feel embarrassed or joyful by tapping into our own store of kinaesthetic knowledge. As the Introduction to this volume shows, even a small word such as "tear" can engage our sensorimotor system in profound ways. And, as the introduction emphasizes, kinesic knowledge can range from pre-reflective to the reflective; it can be both fast and slow (and sometimes, it can be fast and slow at the same time). In his recent book *Thinking with Literature*,

Terence Cave argues that we should not think of the reflective and the pre-reflective as rigidly divided. Reflective knowledge does not simply replace pre-reflective knowledge as our species evolved or as our individual minds developed, he explains. Rather, reflective knowledge can become pre-reflective and vice versa.[5]

Raphael Lyne's 2013 article "The Shakespearean Grasp" has demonstrated that touch and movement, and both action and experience, are important for the handclasp. Tracing in detail the different ways that handclasps can signify in Renaissance culture, Lyne illuminates handclasps in Shakespeare's plays, especially *Coriolanus*, *Measure for Measure*, *Twelfth Night* and *The Comedy of Errors*. He argues that there is "a shared interest, and parallel conclusions, between the two fields" of literature and cognitive science.[6] By showing that both Shakespeare and cognitive theorists are interested in how minds can meet or miss each other through the gestures and touches of the hand, this chapter is founded on a similar acknowledgement of some of the shared stakes of cognitive theory and early modern stagecraft. At the same time, I aim to be aware of the ways in which early modern literature and cognitive theory can speak to each other: perhaps each has something to say that the other had not already thought of.

This chapter will focus on how handclasps function in *Titus Andronicus* and will establish how the early modern handclasp ideally embodies several different meanings: a complex web of metaphors of exchange in dynamic, living play. A cognitive reading helps because it enables us to understand how bodily movements make and contain meaning: they do not just represent thoughts, but shape them. Titus' problem is that he reduces the handclasp to a crude metaphor of exchange, in which his hand is not even an agent of exchange—but an object: "lend me thy hand and I will give thee mine … give his majesty my hand." And, as a result his handclasp is ineffective: it fails to influence Aaron or the emperor; it fails to save his sons, and he ends up brooding on the outskirts of Rome. It is only by tapping into the rich metaphors of thought and emotion associated with the hand that Titus can gain authority again. To handle is to know, to grasp is not just to hold but also to grab something mentally. By harnessing the wider notion of "to handle" (to plan, to scheme, to control), Titus (fully aware of the bitter meaning behind the pun as he has lost one of his physical hands) is able to use his ability to plot and scheme to "lay hands on" (5.2.158) his enemies in revenge. This chapter will also suggest a way that we can think of the touches in this play, and throughout Shakespeare's works, as touching audiences.

Giving with Hands

The early modern handshake is never just a physical movement of two hands together (whatever that might be) but also richly emotional, social and mental. As Carla Mazzio explains, "to touch" in the Renaissance was at once physically to sense the world with one's skin and to have thoughts and emotions that were shaped by the material cultures of this world. She explains, "To feel was, in the Renaissance, a verb used interchangeably with 'to touch', and both verbs implied physical as well as emotional sensation"; "to have 'tact' is to have just the right touch, a manifest sensitivity to one's linguistic and social surrounds."[7] The ideal notion of the handclasp in this era is one in which our physical movements and cognitive (social, emotional, rational, religious, forward-planning) lives are not separate. The cognitive theorist David McNeill has argued that by gesturing, a person is both manifesting and "updating" their cognitive state.[8] That is, the kinesic act and experience of a handshake does not just show people how we are thinking and feeling, it shapes our thoughts and feelings too. And if in practice we attempt to separate the physical movement of the hand from its connection to our brain (as in Titus's crude severed handshake) the handclasp becomes limited, ineffective, a parody of what it ought to be.

So, what does a handshake mean in the early modern era? Giovanni Bonifacio puts it well in his compendium of gestures *L'Arte Dei Cenni* (1612). Bonifacio shows that the gesture of shaking, or giving hands, "dar la mano," was often a metaphorical act of gift-giving. When one takes hands with someone, Bonifacio argues, one is "giving" them something abstract: one's friendship, service, fidelity, love or allegiance, whilst hands themselves are a valuable "gift" from God.[9] As an object of exchange, Titus' dead hand goes too far with this metaphor and as a result destroys the very communal and interactive systems of economic exchange that Titus jokes about. When Titus says "give his majesty my hand," the hand is reduced to an object of exchange, not an agent.

Bonifacio's remarks are echoed in other early modern texts on hands, the most famous of which (as Lyne and Farah Karim-Cooper also explain) is John Bulwer's study *Chirologia* and *Chironomia* (1644): two treatises on hand gestures bound together in the same volume. In this volume, Bulwer categorizes a huge array of hand gestures (from wringing the hands to clapping to raising hands in prayer) and explains their significance in terms of the thoughts that they produce, and are prompted by, in the gesturer's mind. An early modern physician, Bulwer is also credited with writing the first English treatise on sign language, *Philocophus* (1648). Bulwer's preface to *Chirologia … Chironomia* involves a detailed discussion of handclasps that draws on early modern ideas of exchange, and it demonstrates just how richly an ideal act of giving hands is involved in dynamic, multiple metaphoric play.

Dedicating the work to his friend Edward Goldsmith of Gray's Inn,[10] Bulwer states, "having put forth my *Right Hand* in signe of amity to you, and for performance of promise: there remaines nothing (most noble *Chirophilus*) but that you take it in between Yours in token of warranty."[11] This dedication creates a very allusive and polyvalent idea of the hand as figuring in an exchange. In dedicating *Chirologia … Chironomia* to Goldsmith, Bulwer is giving him his hand in the sense of giving him a book called "The Hand" (the preface often roughly and reductively translates *Chironomia*, or "rules of the hand," as "The Hand"). Bulwer is also alluding to the practice of presenting Goldsmith with his flesh and blood hand as an act of friendship. Moreover, he is presenting both book and anatomical hand for Goldsmith to read in both a figurative and a literal act of chiromancy (the subject matter of the book will help Goldsmith to be an even better chiromancer). When Bulwer writes, "you turn'd *Chiromancer*, divining by the lines of *life* and *property*, which appeared fairlie unto you in the first draught, that the Hand would be embraced and kissed by the more intelligent part of the world,"[12] it is unclear whether the "Hand" being kissed here is the book or Bulwer's flesh and blood hand, and whether the "lines" being read are creases in Bulwer's palm or lines of print, ambiguities that perfectly capture the ambiguous playing on the word "Hand" in this preface.

For Bulwer, the hand conveys information not only by being watched as it gestures, but also by being touched, by being given as a gift, by being read as if it were a book by a chiromancer, and by being read as a literal book by the reader. These ideas are perhaps all present in *Titus Andronicus*; with respect to the textuality of the handclasp, for instance, Farah Karim-Cooper suggests that the letter Titus asks the Clown to deliver in Act 4 is "another version of his own hand."[13] Modern cognitive and neurolinguistic texts, such as David McNeill's *Gesture and Thought* and Susan Goldin-Meadow's *Hearing Gesture: How Our Hands Help us Think* reflect the prevalent early modern notion of the hand as the main body part for making signs and for communicating information about a speaker's state of mind. This shared concern makes texts like Bulwer's useful resources for cognitive studies of hand gesture.

Moving beyond the preface, Bulwer sums up the handclasp by saying that it primarily expresses unity of fortunes, love, and minds. It is,

> *An* expression usuall between those who desire to incorporate completely or grow into one, and make a perfect joynt … since they who thus professe communion of good while they willingly embrace each others hand signifie that they are both content that their works shall be common.[14]

And yet Bulwer emphasizes that the handclasp is not just a representation of this "desire to incorporate completely." When he says "signifie" he later qualifies this with a suggestion that there were certain powerful physical properties present in touch that affected, or in McNeill's terminology "updated" the gesturers' cognitive states. Bulwer describes the hand as possessing a "virtue" or power akin to, or consisting in, a magic potion; he uses the word "philtre," which can be read both as a metaphorical assertion that the handclasp's effect on the mind is like a drug and as a literal assumption that there is a chemical substance contained in the hand that affects anyone it touches. Bulwer explains that handshakes are able to bring people together, "hence Physitians the subtile and diligent observers of nature, thinke that there is in the *Hand* a certaine secret and hidden vertue, and a convenient force or philtre to procure *affection*."[15] A handshake is not just a physical movement, nor is it just a metaphor for affection: it *is* affection and it produces affection.

The idea that thought and emotion are embodied in the handshake is present in several important early modern rituals, not least marriage. The widely used Sarum marriage rite, on which the *Book of Common Prayer* is closely based, states that the husband should put the wedding ring on the wife's fourth finger because there was a vein running from there directly to the heart. Touching the sonorous silver ring would thus (via this nerve, with a kind of vibration-effect) remind her at the core of her being of the love that ought to exist between herself and her husband: "And here were put the ring, where, doctors say, there is a certain vein proceeding right to the heart such that the sonority of the silver ring provokes the internal delight that should always exist between the married pair."[16] The *Book of Common Prayer* therefore states that the ring should be placed on "the fowerth finger of the womans left hande."[17] Thus, when Henry VI asks Warwick and Clarence to "join your hands, and with your hands your hearts" (*3 Henry VI* 4.6.39) or Miranda offers Ferdinand her hand in betrothal "with my heart in it" (*The Tempest* 3.1.89–90) they are drawing on this sense that hearts were physically linked during a handclasp. Early modern hands contained hearts; they contained and proffered love and affection.

Titus Andronicus is an early play; with it Shakespeare presents a subverted version of the handclasp before he followed this up with a series of more normative, loving handclasps in plays like *The Tempest* and *Much Ado About Nothing*. Rather than (as Warwick and Clarence in *3 Henry VI* or Miranda in *The Tempest*), giving his heart with a handclasp that enables Aaron to come into contact with the living vein that runs from the hand to the heart, Titus gives Aaron a severed, deadened part of this link to the heart. This is part of the wider way in which *Titus Andronicus* destroys the rich and dynamic metaphorical play that is ideally part of the gesture of taking hands.

So, when we give our hands, we give our hearts and our friendship and receive those of others in return. We open our minds and hearts to be affected by others through touch and we touch others' hands so that we can shape their thoughts and emotions. This is why, as Raleigh and *Etiquette for Dummies* both suggest, a bare, naked hand is necessary for a polite, social handclasp. It is polite to be open to the dynamic, lively touch of the other, rich with metaphorical associations, as we engage in a kinesic interaction with them.

How bare is Titus' hand? Not bare at all. Cut off from his brain and mind, it cannot affect or be affected by any magical philtres. It cannot strike a bargain. It cannot touch Aaron's heart or let Aaron touch his. Titus' subverted "handclasp" with Aaron can even be read as a darkly comedic sign of mistrust. Titus might understandably be reticent about touching the evil Aaron's bare skin with his own, thereby instituting, whether he wants to or not, a bond between them. But, instead of just keeping his gloves on, Titus (in keeping with the extravagantly violent spirit of the whole play) goes one step further and cuts off all his nerves. Shakespeare is testing the limits of embodied social exchanges.

Touching Audiences: A Comparison with *Hamlet*

"If actors knew more about what touches caused in their audiences, they would make use of that information," Lyne suggests, and he captures the way that authors like Shakespeare use touches and "touching" effects on stage to affect audiences in sometimes unpredictable ways, "a dramatist magnifies and merges effects in order to wonder (and wonder at) where they might go."[18] This brings us onto another important aspect of touch in *Titus Andronicus*: "to touch" and "to move" do not just mean the literally kinesic and sensitive touch of the hand, but also the ability of what we witness onstage to "touch" or "move" us emotionally: to make us feel something, to stir us.

This wider notion of "touching" is something that Tamora is well aware of. As she revenges herself on Titus by removing his ability to clasp hands, she makes it clear that she is interested in touching him in the wider sense of harming the core of his being, affecting him, making him feel desperate, isolated and bitter, "Titus, I have touch'd thee to the quick" (4.4.35), Tamora gloats as she arrives to revel in his ultimate grief-stricken madness. Deploying the word "touch" to mean "harm," and using it to cut Titus off from society rather than build bonds, Tamora perverts the empathetic, mutual cognitive exchanges that touch can usually achieve.

Here, it is worthwhile comparing *Titus Andronicus* to a later play, *Hamlet*, where light touches touch the audience particularly strongly. In the final duel in *Hamlet*, Laertes states that he will give only the very tip of his sword the merest "touch" of poison, "I'll touch my point/With this contagion, that if I gall him slightly,/It may be death" (4.7.146–8). Laertes imagines simply chafing or breaking the surface of Hamlet's skin (two contemporary meanings of "to gall.")[19] He further stresses the lack of energetic violence needed in this final duel, stating that Hamlet may "be but scratch'd withal" and he will die (4.7.146). This careful framing has a significant effect on the way that stage violence in *Hamlet* is imagined by audiences, readers and actors. It also has an effect on the way that Hamlet and Laertes' final duel can be acted, because it relieves the actors from the need to simulate violent, bloody mortal combat.

This perhaps makes the stage violence in *Hamlet* more able to touch an audience—because it looks more realistic. Unlike kisses and handshakes, which can be performed on stage with as much skin contact as we expect from "real" kisses and handshakes off stage, stage punches and sword thrusts often involve encouraging the viewer to imagine bodily contact that in fact is not enacted. Staged fights-to-the-death are usually moments when actors' and characters' intentions diverge. Whilst one or both characters are trying their hardest to harm the other, the actors are trying hard not to really hurt each other at all. The gap between actors' bodies as characters supposedly make violent contact with each other becomes a widening gap between fiction and reality. When audiences can see actors slapping their own wrists instead of each other's faces, or smacking swords onto the stage-floor as their opponent pretends that the sword has wounded them, the fiction that the action on stage involves two people wounding and killing each other is punctured and empathizing with the characters may be more difficult.

Terry King, fight director for Gregory Doran's 2008 RSC *Hamlet*, argues that, compared to the mass brawls of Shakespeare's histories, the duel in *Hamlet* is set up so that it has to be particularly realistic and convincing as it involves just two opponents:

> The biggest challenge in *Hamlet* is that there is nothing to distract attention from the fights. Arranging big fight scenes with lots of people on stage does present its own problems, but it also means that the swordplay doesn't have to be very clever, because your eyes are constantly being pulled all around the stage. In Hamlet there is a lot of focus on just two people fighting, they are the centre of attention.[20]

The device of the poisoned foil means that Laertes and Hamlet's final duel can bear this scrutiny, as it is not difficult to make a slight graze look realistic. This device both acknowledges and masks the difference between actors and characters because a slight graze can be simulated realistically without endangering the actors. Thus, during this stage fight there is little divergence between what the actors are doing and what they appear to be doing; both actors and characters are fencing and only touching each other lightly.

When Osric notes "a very palpable hit" (5.2.281), he redoubles the idea of touching inherent in "hit" as "palpable" derives from Latin *palpabilis* (that which may be touched). Osric's word "palpable" also extends the idea of touching from a literal "hit" to a touch that is imagined, as "palpable" also had the wider figurative sense of something that is sensed or felt with the mind.[21] Vocabulary of touching and smelling was often used to indicate mental influence in the early modern era and in particular was a common way of envisaging the ways that people could be influenced by each other at the theatre: anti-theatricalists used imagery of poison, drugs and infection to demonstrate this. Stephen Gosson, for instance, writes of on-stage kisses, "as the stinge of *Phalangion* spreadeth her poyson through euery vaine, when no hurt is seene; so amorous gesture, strikes to the heart when no skinne is raced."[22] Kathryn Banks' chapter in this volume is invaluable for shedding further light on ideas of knowing through, or as, taste and smell. Her work suggests, perhaps, that Gosson's images of ingested poison are not accidental. Rather, via the framework TO INGEST is TO KNOW, they demonstrate that this wicked knowledge that Gosson envisages emanating from theatrical productions is something that inhabits and infects us bodily.

Laertes links the touch of his sword to olfaction and airborne contamination by describing the poison as a "contagion," which derives from the Latin *con-tangere*, (to touch together). *Hamlet* is the first recorded usage for both the literal and figurative meanings of "contagion": a disease passed on by touching, or a pernicious mental influence. The Oxford English Dictionary lists Laertes' use of "contagion" to mean "poison" as the first usage of this concrete meaning of contagion, and Hamlet's image of hell "breath[ing] forth … contagion" from graves (3.2.389–90) as the first figurative usage. "Contagion" could also simply mean "influence."[23] When Laertes states that he will merely "touch" the "point" of his sword with "contagion," the word "contagion" completely overturns the minimal, highly localized physical contact implied by "touch" and "point" (which conjure up an image of Laertes just dabbing the sharp point of a sword with some poison). The word "contagion" turns this dabbing gesture into an action that suggests a spreading infection that has a broad effect that is both physical and psychological. As well as spreading to infect Hamlet, this contagion spreads to infect Claudius and Laertes himself when Hamlet turns the sword against them. Moreover, the sight of this stage violence has the power potentially to "infect" audience's minds with violent, fearful or aggressive thoughts. Poised at a crucial moment in a play where language becomes violent and tangible in unprecedented ways, Laertes' sword is tipped with a particularly theatrical poison, which persuasively influences audiences to imagine that they are seeing a fight to the death.

Even a light touch onstage can "touch" an audience if it resonates with the metaphors that we have (kinesically) learned. Laertes' foil striking Hamlet and Titus' severed hand slumping into Aaron's grasp can stir us with horror, wonder, fear, and dark laughter. This motif of light touches is, as Marjorie O'Rourke Boyle has shown, part of a wider Renaissance interest in "delicate" touches between humans, and between the human and the divine.[24]

There is no denying that the moment when Titus' hand is severed in *Titus Andronicus* has the power to touch audiences. The (failed) touch of Titus' severed hand with Aaron's living one moves outwards and touches audiences with "wonder" (as Lyne describes), shock and disgust. In 2006 at the Globe, director Lucy Bailey concentrated on making the scenes of severed hands as horrifying as possible by using realistic dummy hands filled with false blood and tubes hidden in actors' sleeves that spurted constant and copious supplies of even more false blood.[25] Dominic Dromgoole's Artistic Director's speech at the end of the 2006 run mentioned the spate of faintings as a highlight of the season, the successful creation of a lasting image of the hand offered and severed.[26] Rashid Razaq wrote for the *Evening Standard* on 5 May 2006 of "Theatregoers Passing Out Over Gory Scenes at the Globe," and Richard Stott focused for *The Sunday Mirror* on 11 June on "first aiders and wheelchairs" being brought in to help people who fainted ("It's No Holds Bard.").

There have been more surprising reactions, though, which may indeed make us "wonder at" the power of severed hands and failed or absent touches in this play. Vivien Leigh's Lavinia in Peter Brook's production at the Shakespeare Memorial Theatre in 1955 elicited gasps from the audience as she appeared in an exquisite gown with red ribbons streaming from her wrists. According to the actress Janet Suzman, these audiences were shocked not because the scene was so gory but "because [Leigh] was so beautiful."[27] Her glamorous appearance created such an iconic image that other productions (e.g. Yukio Ninagawa's in 2006) deploying this ribbon-device tend to be seen as referencing or echoing Brook's definitive use of it. Rich in metaphor, the handshake shocks us when it is not performed properly. We feel the difference between practice and ideal, and we become aware of the way that touch is not just physical but more widely cognitive.

Conclusion

Titus Andronicus invites Shakespeare's audiences to deploy their kinesic intelligence in understanding exchanges of hands that are at once embodied and metaphorical and which shift between these two poles in surprising and gruesome ways. Early modern handshakes are certainly bodily movements. But they are not just that: they are also richly metaphorical moments, and we understand them through these metaphors. Metaphors are in dynamic play here as two bodies interact: bargains and friendships are exchanged, minds and emotions are moved with and by hands, and hearts and hands are touched simultaneously. The subverted handshake that we have looked at in *Titus Andronicus* is shocking not just because it is horrific and painful but also because it crudely reduces the usual rich metaphoric life of the handshake as an interaction of two agents (where hearts, hands, minds, thoughts, loves, friendships are in lively interaction) to a crude bargain.

This moment is shocking because of the gore and pain we imagine it involves. But Titus' joke about giving Aaron his hand can also shock us because using handclasps to make friends, bargain sincerely or marry is important to us. Titus' hand is not the richly metaphorical agent of exchange that is the ideal we see in Bulwer's treatise, it is no longer a gateway to Titus' rich cognitive life but simply an object of exchange. Dead flesh, can only be exchanged for dead flesh: Titus' two sons are not returned to him alive (as he hopes them, "jewels purchas'd at an easy price" 3.1.198) but dead. His hand itself is, as the messenger who brings it states, "in scorn to thee sent back" (3.1.237).

Notes

1. Walter Raleigh, *The History of the World*, 2nd ed. (London: William Stansby, 1617), Fff2r.
2. Henry Siddons, *Practical Illustrations of Rhetorical Gesture and Action Adapted to the English Drama from a Work on the Subject by M Engel*, 2nd ed. (London: Sherwood, Neely, and Jones, 1822), 164.
3. Sue Fox, *Etiquette for Dummies* (Hoboken, NJ: Wiley, 2011), 150.
4. Guillemette Bolens, *The Style of Gestures: Embodiment and Cognition in Literary Narrative* (Baltimore: Johns Hopkins, 2012), 1–3.
5. "Any notion of a radical cleavage between unconscious and conscious (pre-reflective and reflective) mental functioning runs counter to the fundamental premise of embodied cognition, namely that all cognitive processes operate on a gradient between sensorimotor perceptions and responses on the one hand and so-called higher-order conceptual activities on the other," *Thinking with Literature: Towards a Cognitive Criticism* (Oxford: Oxford University Press, 2016), 30.
6. Raphael Lyne, "The Shakespearean Grasp," *Cambridge Quarterly* 42, no. 1 (2013): 61. Farah Karim-Cooper has recently published a book-length study of the hand, *The Hand on the Shakespearean Stage: Gesture, Touch and the Spectacle of Dismemberment* (London: Bloomsbury, 2016). Though she does not use cognitive theory, Karim-Cooper explores the tension between ideal and actual practice when it comes to social gestures, explaining that "the way hands moved or were accounted for in performance forms a polysemous system incorporating a combination of instinctive, everyday and more formal or iconic gestures [...] gestures moved between all and each of these extremes depending on the various contexts in which they occur." She also examines tactility and the way that the grasping, touching hands of audience members were a significant part of the theatrical experience. *The Hand*, 42, 115.

7. Carla Mazzio, *The Inarticulate Renaissance* (Philadelphia: Pennsylvania University Press, 2009), 180, 214.
8. David McNeill, *Gesture and Thought* (Chicago: Chicago University Press, 2005), 91–2.
9. Giovanni Bonifacio, *L'Arte Dei Cenni* (Venice: Francisco Grossi, 1616, first published 1612), 290. [my translation].
10. There are two Edward Goldsmiths in the register of admissions to Gray's Inn in the seventeenth century: one in 1621 and one in 1624, John Foster, *The Register of Admissions to Gray's Inn, 1521–1889* (London: The Hansard Publishing Union, 1889), 781, 823.
11. John Bulwer, "Chirologia" in *Chirologia…Chironomia* (London: Thomas Harper, 1644), A4^{r}.
12. Bulwer, *Chirologia*, A2^{v}.
13. Karim-Cooper, *The Hand on the Shakespearean Stage*, 3.
14. Bulwer, *Chirologia*, H7^{r-v}.
15. Bulwer, *Chirologia*, I2^{v}-I3^{r}.
16. "Ibique dimittat annulum. Quia in medico est quaedam vena procedens vsque ad cor et in sonoritate argenti designatur interna dilecto, quae semper inter eos debet esse recens," Clement Maydeston, ed., *Ordinale Sarum* [facsimile] (London: Wynkyn de Worde, 1508), 27.
17. Thomas Cranmer et al., *The Book of the Common Prayer* (London: Edward Whytchurche, 1549), 30^{r}.
18. Lyne, "The Shakespearean Grasp," 61.
19. O.E.D., "gall," v^{1}, 1, 3.
20. Terry King, in *Programme, Hamlet, by William Shakespeare,* directed by Gregory Doran (Royal Shakespeare Company, 2008), 4^{r}.
21. O.E.D., "palpable," *adj*, 1, 3–4.
22. Stephen Gosson, *Playes Confuted in Five Actions* (London: for Thomas Gosson, 1582), G5^{r}.
23. O.E.D., "contagion," *n*, 3 b, c, 4.
24. For a discussion of the "delicate" touch of God, for instance, see Marjorie O'Rourke Boyle, *Senses of Touch: Human Dignity and Deformity from Michelangelo to Calvin* (Leiden: Brill, 1998), 202.
25. For instance, when Titus' hand was severed, he laid his hand on a chopping block then hid it in his sleeve, and a false hand filled with blood popped up from inside the block, which Aaron then hacked at. "Fight Notes 2," *Titus Andronicus, by William Shakespeare*, directed by Lucy Bailey, Globe Theatre, 2006, Globe Theatre Archive. Prompt Book, *Titus Andronicus*, by William Shakespeare, directed by Lucy Bailey, Globe Theatre, 2006, Globe Theatre Archive.
26. Dominic Dromgoole, *Artistic Director's Speech*, 2006, Globe Theatre Archive, London.
27. Gregory Doran and Anthony Sher, *Woza Shakespeare: Titus Andronicus in South Africa* (London: Methuen, 1996), 218.

Bibliography

Bolens, Guillemette. *The Style of Gestures: Embodiment and Cognition in Literary Narrative*. Baltimore: Johns Hopkins, 2012.

Bonifacio, Giovanni. *L'Arte Dei Cenni*. Venice: Francisco Grossi, 1616 first published 1612.

Bulwer, John. *Chirologia…Chironomia*. London: Thomas Harper, 1644.

Cave, Terence. *Thinking with Literature: Towards a Cognitive Criticism*. Oxford: Oxford University Press, 2016.

Cranmer, Thomas, et al. *The Book of the Common Prayer*. London: Edward Whytchurche, 1549.

Doran, Gregory, and Anthony Sher. *Woza Shakespeare: Titus Andronicus in South Africa*. London: Methuen, 1996.

Dromgoole, Dominic. *Artistic Director's Speech*. London: Globe Theatre Archive, 2006.

Fight Notes 2. *Titus Andronicus, by William Shakespeare*. Directed by Lucy Bailey. Globe Theatre. London: Globe Theatre Archive, 2006.

Foster, John. *The Register of Admissions to Gray's Inn, 1521–1889*. London: The Hansard Publishing Union, 1889.

Fox, Sue. *Etiquette for Dummies*. Hoboken, NJ: Wiley, 2011.

Goldin-Meadow, Susan. *Hearing Gesture: How Our Hands Help Us Think*. Cambridge, MA: Harvard University Press, 2003.

Gosson, Stephen. *Playes Confuted in Five Actions*. London: Thomas Gosson, 1582.

Karim-Cooper, Farah. *The Hand on the Shakespearean Stage: Gesture, Touch and the Spectacle of Dismemberment*. London: Bloomsbury, 2016.

King, Terry. *Programme. Hamlet, by William Shakespeare*. Directed by Gregory Doran. Royal Shakespeare Company, 2008.

Lyne, Raphael. The Shakespearean Grasp. *Cambridge Quarterly* 42, no. 1 (2013): 38–61.

Maydeston, Clement, ed. *Ordinale Sarum* [facsimile]. London: Wynkyn de Worde, 1508.

Mazzio, Carla. *The Inarticulate Renaissance*. Philadelphia: Pennsylvania University Press, 2009.

McNeill, David. *Gesture and Thought*. Chicago: Chicago University Press, 2005.

O'Rourke Boyle, Marjorie. *Senses of Touch: Human Dignity and Deformity from Michelangelo to Calvin*. Leiden: Brill, 1998.

Prompt Book. *Titus Andronicus*, by William Shakespeare, directed by Lucy Bailey, Globe Theatre. London: Globe Theatre Archive, 2006

Raleigh, Walter. *The History of the World*. 2nd ed. London: William Stansby, 1617.

Siddons, Henry. *Practical Illustrations of Rhetorical Gesture and Action Adapted to the English Drama from a Work on the Subject by M Engel*. 2nd ed. London: Sherwood, Neely, and Jones, 1822.

CHAPTER 9

"Cabin'd, Cribb'ed, Confin'd": Images of Thwarted Motion in *Macbeth*

Mary Thomas Crane

When looking for kinesic effects in literature for this volume, I noticed a powerful nexus of images in Shakespeare's *Macbeth* that conveyed a sense of entrapment, suffocation and thwarted movement, and which, it seemed to me, might prompt a reader or audience member to view Macbeth's violent actions with some level of understanding or sympathy—perhaps explaining how we remain interested in following the progress of a serial murderer. But as I worked on writing the essay, I retained a nagging dissatisfaction with my reading of *Macbeth* because I was haunted by a question that I could not immediately answer: how would my focus on the kinesic effects of these images differ from a new critical focus on any pattern of imagery in the play? If I were to leave out all reference to kinesis, simulation, or embodiment, and were to argue (as I might have done in the 1990s) that these images referred to various systems of ideology in which Macbeth was trapped, and that they therefore explained his turn to violence, what would my argument be missing? Or, to put the question another way, what would a focus on kinesis add to that kind of traditional close reading?

M.T. Crane (✉)
Boston College, Chestnut Hill, MA, USA

K. Banks, T. Chesters (eds.), *Movement in Renaissance Literature*, Cognitive Studies in Literature and Performance,
https://doi.org/10.1007/978-3-319-69200-5_9

Thinking about this problem, and reading articles on *Macbeth*, I was reminded that Cleanth Brooks's seminal New Critical essay on the play in his book *The Well Wrought Urn* begins with a section discussing the ways in which poetic images might be understood and discussed. Brooks seems to be working out the terms of what Wimsatt and Beardsley, writing in 1946, had called the "intentional fallacy," the New Critical dictum that "the desire or intention of the author is neither available nor desirable as a standard for judging the success of a work of literary art."[1] Brooks begins his chapter on images of children and clothing in *Macbeth* by alluding to contemporary "debate about the proper limits of metaphor," going on to distinguish between images that seem consciously intended by the author (Donne's compass in his poem "A Valediction: Forbidding Mourning") and imagery (in a style associated with Shakespeare) that upon analysis seems patterned and significant, but which the author seems not to have consciously intended. He describes Donne's images as "self-conscious and witty" and Shakespeare's as "spontaneous comparisons struck out in the heat of composition, and not carefully articulated, self-conscious conceits at all."[2] Upon reflection, however, he discovers that Donne also makes use of "abrupt and succinct comparisons."

In the introduction to the volume, Brooks had already determined that "the language of poetry is the language of paradox," identifying his method of close reading as a process of coming to understand the "underlying paradox" that he argues necessarily lies behind every poem.[3] His reading of *Macbeth* proceeds by showing how what seem to be unconscious (and initially illogical) images can be demonstrated by the critic to be part of a thematically meaningful (paradoxical) pattern. Thus, passages that initially seem to make no sense (how can a "naked new-born babe" be capable of "striding the blast"?) are shown to be part of a pattern of images of children and clothing that express the paradoxes at the heart of the play: "pity is like the naked babe, the most sensitive and helpless thing: yet, almost as soon as the comparison is announced, the symbol of weakness begins to turn into a symbol of strength."[4]

Brooks ultimately leaves open the question of whether Shakespeare intentionally created the pattern of images that he has traced. He simply notes that the "symbols" of children and clothing in the play "demonstrate how far the conscious or unconscious symbolism could take [Shakespeare]." But if the author's conscious intention is not necessary as an imagined condition for meaningful imagery, the critic is presented as fully conscious in his logical parsing of the "symbols" present in the poem.

Brooks the critic translates these symbols for us, explaining what they mean, bringing them up against each other until they generate the logical paradoxes that he feels are central to poetic expression.

Interestingly, though, it is possible to identify a rudimentary kinesic component to Brooks's own language, which may play a role in predisposing readers to accept his argument. In characterizing the act of poetic composition, Brooks caricatures the "self-conscious" poet who intends all of his poetic effects as "not a fervent poet but a preternaturally cold and self-conscious monster."[5] With this coldness, he contrasts a poet writing "in the heat of composition," whose imagery (in Coleridge's terms) involves "the rapid flow, the quick change" and "intellectual vigor."[6] Shakespeare's imagery of children in *Macbeth* is not "a rather stiff and mechanical allegory" but rather "flexible," possessing a "flexibility that must amaze the reader." Similarly, Macbeth and Lady Macbeth are shown to be coldly unpitying—the naked babe represents "that which should be clothed and warmed." Macbeth's "overbrittle rationalism" is defeated by the paradox that "pity is strong because of its weakness."[7] Overly self-conscious authors, and insufficiently empathetic tyrants are both portrayed as stiff and cold; vigorous poets and their poetic language are flexible and warm.

Brooks's essay raises questions about the relationship between the effects of literary images and the consciousness of both poet and reader that cognitive literary theory is better able to answer than could New Criticism, since it offers a more nuanced sense of the relationship between unconscious and conscious mental processes, viewing them as existing on a continuum rather than in opposition to each other. In the introduction to this volume, Kathryn Banks and Timothy Chesters describe the analysis of kinesic images as involving both pre-conscious and conscious elements, in which "what begins as a pre-conscious response on a first reading of the poem is likely to be expanded, into a series of more deliberate rehearsals, as we model in more reflective and conscious ways a wide variety of candidate movements."[8] In their view, building on the work of Ellen Spolsky and Guillemette Bolens, "kinesic intelligence" involves both the pre-conscious motor resonance activated by images that involve simulated movement and also conscious critical reflection on the significance of those images. Terence Cave, in *Thinking with Literature*, suggests that "there is a perceivable continuity, an indivisible gradient between bodily response and cognitive analysis," so that a "cognitive reading" of a literary text would "seek to uncover the hidden work of rapid inferencing and on-the-wing construction of meaning" that happens as we read.[9]

The images of thwarted motion in *Macbeth* may raise a slightly different version of these questions about the relationship between conscious and pre-conscious images. If pre-conscious motor resonance exists on a continuum with conscious awareness of it and critical reflection upon it, do both ends of the continuum impact the reader in the same way? It seems possible that in the case of *Macbeth*, the stage of pre-conscious resonance with imagery of movement in the play might be at odds with an analysis that brings it to consciousness and calls attention to it. The critical history of the play reveals that critical readers have tended to subsume the imagery of thwarted movement (if they notice it at all) into a dominant image pattern of headlong speed. These readers associate speed with wilful ambition, and interpret Macbeth's violent headlong rush into the future as the way the play signals his moral failing. Harold Toliver, in an essay published in 1965, argued that Macbeth "destroys the present in reaching ahead for the future."[10] In these readings, images of thwarted movement are not noticed, or are associated with the moral consequences of Macbeth's overleaping, which, in Toliver's words, leads to "a smothering of sequential order and hierarchy in private, 'horrible imaginings.'"[11] I will argue that the imagery of smothering, choking and balking is pervasive throughout the play, precedes and contributes to causing Macbeth's ambitious overleaping, and that it may work to elicit a sympathetic identification with Macbeth that critics may repress as they focus on condemnation of him. Critics who emphasize rapid movement in the play base their argument on factors other than kinesic imagery, including the brevity of the play and many of its scenes, abstract references to time, and a relatively few references to the need for instantaneous action.[12] The language of smothering and thwarted movement, on the other hand, is conveyed primarily through resonant images of physical experience. We need to ask why so many critics ignore or downplay a set of powerful kinesic images in favor of largely abstract references that suggest their opposite. Could this be because motor resonance leads to feeling rather than judgment, and because judging Macbeth is a more comfortable critical position than empathizing with him?

Shakespeare's *Macbeth* is famous for its troubled history in the theatre, and it has troubled critics as well. Stephen Greenblatt has asked whether the play is, through its depiction of witchcraft, complicit in the persecution of women that happened during the infamous witch trials of the period. Greenblatt ultimately absolves the play of explicitly encouraging the murder of women, but he cites critics like Peter Stallybrass and Janet Adelman who have also seen the play as representing and perhaps encouraging a misogynist fear of powerful women.[13] If kinesic imagery works on an unconscious level to motivate an audience to share the feelings of entrapment and frustration that lead Macbeth to turn to violence, it might represent another morally questionable aspect of the play. Certainly the anti-theatrical tracts of the period believed that plays had pernicious hidden powers over audiences, so it seems possible that kinesis might provide a modern name for this power.

Cognitive approaches to theatrical performance have fruitfully explored the ways in which concepts like "mirror neurons"—which fire as if the subject were actually enacting motions and gestures that are seen—can contribute to our understanding of theatre as a fully embodied experience.[14] But the experience of an early modern play performed on the relatively bare platform stage of the Globe notoriously depends as much on verbal scene-painting as on concrete movement, gesture and prop. We only know that we are in Illyria, in the dark, witnessing the dawn, or in the forest, because characters tell us so. It stands to reason, then, that the imagistic richness of Shakespearean drama offers another traceable effect on the audience that contributes to the phenomenological footprint of the plays, in this case images of choking, suffocation and balked movement help an audience to experience Macbeth's frustration at his thwarted ambition, and to buy in to his succession of violent actions, until in the end he also succumbs to self-defeating stasis.

Throughout the play, clusters of images represent movement being prevented by atmospheric effects, internal humoral conditions, and by characters and events imagined as physical barriers or confining enclosures.[15] A number of critics have noticed that Shakespeare's *Macbeth* places particular emphasis on disturbances of the elements and humours: bubbled air, penetrating winds, thickened blood. Stuart Clark emphasizes early modern interest in the power of air to create optical illusions, and early modern beliefs that demonic forces could be a product of or could manipulate these illusions.[16] Werner Habicht similarly traces the relationship between kinds of air and theatrical illusion.[17] Mary Floyd-Wilson has argued that the play is pervasively concerned with the geo-humoral conditions that made Scottish people particularly "passible," or vulnerable to influential penetration by external environmental (sometimes preternatural) forces.[18]

Shakespeare's *Macbeth* also takes place in a world where directed or teleological movement is pervasively blocked or disturbed. The play is full of powerfully physical images of matter that is thickened, and that chokes or strangles. The witches, as Stuart Clark has argued, are plausibly an optical illusion created by thickened air. Human beings in this atmosphere find their expected or desired movements balked and occluded. Persistent language of "overleaping" and "overtaking" traces failed human attempts to overcome the play's suffocating stasis (rather than, as many critics suggest, Macbeth's wilful speed). Shakespeare's *Macbeth* suggests that a context for the pervasive evil of the play is natural and not necessarily supernatural, a function of an environment that stifles human ambition and creativity.

Many critics have traced patterns of imagery in the play—clothing, blood, darkness, children—which, they have argued, show up the moral bankruptcy of the Macbeths and to some extent of the aristocratic warrior culture they inhabit.[19] In contrast, the play's images of stasis, choking, suffocation and overleaping work to give naturalistic explanations of and gain sympathy for the actions of the witches and of Macbeth and Lady Macbeth who inhabit a universe where atmospheric, humoral, and social conditions are unpredictable, untrustworthy, and block expected teleologies. The play's cultural imaginary, focused on hierarchy, clothing, and natural bonds of kinship and nurturance, constitutes an unsuccessful attempt to counter its unruly natural conditions.

The play opens with the witches who identify the atmospheric conditions that support them, conditions of thickened or bubbled air through which the movement of light and objects is distorted: they are able to "hover through the fog and filthy air." Stuart Clark has traced early modern discussions of the ability of air to carry "visual (and aural) images of all things, carrying them into the bodies of men and women through their pores to create dreams," so that "air was thus an element of sleights and tricks, not one of transparency and truth."[20] Banquo and Macbeth both explain the witches as creatures of air: "The earth hath bubbles, as the water has,/And these are of them" (1.3.79–80); "they made themselves air, into which they vanished" (1.5.4–5).[21] There may be a suggestion that vapours from their bubbling cauldron, full of "gruel thick and slab" (4.1.32) creates the conditions in which they can appear.[22] The witches are famously limited in their agency: they can create windy conditions for the pilot but "his bark cannot be lost."[23] They are creatures of disrupted motion, but are stymied in their power to effect change. They may be able to "look into the seeds of time and say which grain will grow and which will not," but it is not clear to what extent their meddling has the power to alter this teleology.

The witches' primary power seems at least initially to lie in their ability to halt Macbeth in his tracks, to startle and arrest him. When the witches suddenly appear to Macbeth and Banquo out of the fog and proclaim their surprising prophecies, Banquo asks Macbeth "why do you start?" and describes him twice in the lines that follow as "rapt." (1.3.152, 158, 256).[24] In Macbeth's letter to his wife, he describes his own reaction to their prophecy: "whiles I stood rapt in the wonder of it" (1.5.349), and when Macbeth ponders the implications of the news that he has been named Thane of Cawdor in an aside, Banquo comments "look how our partner's rapt." (1.3.144). "Rapt" is derived from the Latin participle "raptus" or seized, with uses in English suggesting that someone's consciousness has been seized or transported, leading to "a state of rapture, enthrallment, or fascination" (OED).[25] "Enthrall" and "fascinate" both suggest the use of magic to seize the will of another, but Macbeth also views their intervention as a physical stoppage, asking them "why/Upon this blasted heath you stop our way." (1.3.77) and wishing, when they have vanished, "would they had stayed!" (1.3.82). Banquo, on the other hand, is not similarly halted or rapt at their words, nor does he wish them to remain.

While Banquo notes Macbeth's "rapt" appearance, Macbeth himself describes the inner causes of his arrested state. His "function is smothered in surmise," (1.3.142) as he imagines an inner state of suffocation corresponding with the outer fog and filthy air associated with the witches. The image of Duncan's murder makes his "seated heart knock at my ribs/ Against the use of nature," as if his heart were trying to escape its entrapment within his body. While the arresting power of the witches is initially associated with either toxic atmospheric conditions, or with some sort of supernatural power, Macbeth now begins to imagine attempts to escape from the rapt state of inner turmoil that they have induced by taking some unnatural action. When he attempts to reassure himself at the end of this speech, he does so by imagining that he need not take action to escape the forces that have seemingly entrapped him, since the prophecy may come true "without my stir" (1.3.146).

Lady Macbeth initially links her own ability to help Macbeth overcome "all that impedes thee from the golden round" with a disruption of the humoral flow within her own body: "Make thick my blood,/Stop up th'access and passage to remorse,/That no compunctious visitings of nature/Shake my fell purpose." (1.5.44–46). Ironically, though, as critics have pointed out, this humoral thickening would also disrupt her reproductive faculty and contribute to the balking of Macbeth's dynastic ambitions, the natural movement of the crown from father to son.[26] Ultimately her thickened blood results in an "infected mind," and she is trapped in the obsessive, repetitive motion of hand washing, until her suicide cuts short her life.

Just as the thick air associated with the witches causes an internal "smothering" in Macbeth, Lady Macbeth imagines that her thickened blood has an atmospheric corollary: "come, thick night,/And pall thee in the dunnest smoke of hell" (1.5.46–47). Before the murder of the king, morally good characters like Banquo perceive the air in Scotland as "delicate," or like Duncan feel that "the air/Nimbly and sweetly recommends itself/Unto our gentle senses" (1.6.10, 1–2). After the murder, characters note that "dark night strangles the traveling lamp" (Ross, 2.4.7), that "light thickens" and "good things of day begin to droop and drowse" (Macbeth, 3.2.52). The murder itself is also associated with inner humoral thickenings and smotherings. In order to get at Duncan, the Macbeths plan to get his grooms drunk, so that "memory the warder of the brain/ Shall be a fume," and "in swinish sleep/Their drenched natures lies as in a death" (1.7.67–69). Macbeth informs Donalbain of his father's murder with another image of humoral blockage: "The spring, the head, the fountain of your blood/Is stopped, the very source of it is stopped" (2.3.91–92).

The political world of the play is also characterized by stasis and blocked movement.[27] The opening battle is initially described as stuck: "doubtful it stood,/As two spent swimmers that do cling together/And choke their art" (1.2.7–9). "Choking" here may link the stymied battle once again with the fog and filthy air conjured up by the witches. Macbeth brings welcome relief when he literally cuts his way through the battle and dismembers Macdonwald, although his sword "which smok'd with bloody execution" (1.2.18) reminds us that he also is a creature of the filthy air. The persistent doubling language of the play mirrors this sense of stasis: what Macdonwald has lost, Macbeth has won. They balance each other out.

Duncan initially describes his desire to reward Macbeth in terms of motion: "thou art so far before,/That swiftest wing of recompense is slow/To overtake thee" (1.4.16–18). His decision to thwart expectation and name his son Malcolm as his heir involves another kind of overtaking: Macbeth's expected rise to power is overtaken by Malcolm. Macbeth not surprisingly describes this as a barrier to his own upward movement: "that is a step/On which I must fall down, or else o'er leap,/For in my way it lies." (1.4.48–50). The soliloquy at the beginning of act 1 scene 7 in which he convinces himself not to kill Duncan is also full of images of balked or interrupted motion: Macbeth speaks of wanting to "trammel up the consequence," for this "blow" to be "the be-all and the end-all—here." He twice echoes his earlier image of jumping over an obstacle, but now in forms that represent motion that doesn't make clear forward progress: he would "jump the life to come," and his "vaulting ambition" "o'erleaps itself." Air, the medium of strange motion in the play, reappears in the famously incongruous image of the "new-born babe,/Striding the blast, or heaven's cherubin, hors'd/Upon the sightless couriers of the air" that will "blow the horrid deed in every eye,/That tears shall drown the wind." Duncan's virtues, like the witches, can create a powerful wind that will reveal his murder, but even here that movement of the wind will be "drowned"—another image of smothering—by his mourners' tears. All of this seeming movement—jumping, leaping, blasting—comes to nothing.

If up until the murder of Duncan the play depicts Macbeth as trapped and smothered by external forces, it shifts after that point to associating Macbeth himself with suffocation and impeded motion, an alteration in kinesic energy that may prepare an audience to shift its sympathies away from Macbeth. After Macbeth kills Duncan, he increasingly sees his movement toward his desired goal as blocked, and even self-blocking, often in terms of things getting stuck: "I had most need of blessing and 'amen' stuck in my throat" (2.2.30), "our fears in Banquo stick deep" (3.1.49). Macbeth explains his seemingly rash murder of the grooms as involving the overcoming of an internal blockage: "th' expedition of my violent love/Outrun the pauser, reason" (2.3.110–11). Banquo's threat to Macbeth—the offspring that will inherit the throne after Macbeth—is seen in terms of "wrenching" the sceptre away from Macbeth, his line of progeny disrupted by an "unlineal hand." Macbeth reacts to the news that Banquo's son, Fleance, has escaped the murderers who killed his father by describing another state of self-entrapment: "now I am cabin'd, cribb'd, confin'd, bound in/To saucy doubts and fears" (3.4.23–4). The appearance of Banquo's ghost is seen by Macbeth as an interruption of the natural teleology of things: "the time had been/That when the brains were out, the man would die/And there an end; but now they rise again" (3.4.77–9). At this juncture he sees himself trapped in a kind of stasis that recalls that of the two spent swimmers of act 1: "I am in blood/Stepp'd in so far that, should I wade no more,/Returning were as tedious as go o'er" (3.5.135). Macbeth has gone from imagining himself leaping over obstacles, chopping his way through the battlefield, to seeing his progress as a slog, where both going forward and going back are equally tedious. He understands, at least, that he is most confined by his own paranoid fear.

When Macbeth again consults the witches in 4.1, in an attempt to gain reassurance that his intended trajectory will continue, he is met with several prophecies involving unnatural motion: he will only be killed by someone not of woman born, and not until trees move on their own. On the other hand Banquo's line will not be interrupted, but will "Stretch out even to th' crack of doom" (4.1.117). Macbeth then echoes Duncan's language about overtaking: "the flightly purpose never is o'ertook/Unless the deed go with it" (4.1.145–6). Deeds, like recompense, are hopelessly belated unless thought and action are collapsed: "be it thought and done." However, his desire to speed up the achievement of his purpose falls back soon enough into a sense of purposeless tedium: "tomorrow and tomorrow and tomorrow/Creeps in this petty pace from day to day" (5.4.19–20).

Toward the end of the play, both his opponents and Macbeth himself feel that Scotland is in need of purgation in order to free itself from some form of internal blockage. Caithness and Angus, both in league with Malcolm, note that Macbeth is no longer able to confine himself: "he cannot buckle his distemper'd cause/Within the belt of rule" (5.2.15–16). Now his crimes, "the secret murders sticking on his hands," are what impede him, and the rebels view themselves as "the med'cine of the sickly weal" whose blood will be "our country's purge" (5.2.27, 28). At the same time, Macbeth asks the doctor to cure both Lady Macbeth and Scotland by purging, treating his wife with "some sweet oblivious antidote" that will "cleanse the stuff'd bosom of that perilous stuff/Which weighs upon the heart" (4.2.43–5). He also asks for "a purgative drug" that would "scour these English hence" and rid the country of those fighting against him (4.2.55–6).

For both sides, this purge takes the form of yet more violence, which remains the only alternative to blockage and stasis that the characters can imagine. Macbeth calls on the "intrenchant air" (5.8.9) as proof of his invulnerability, but the trees do walk, and Macduff was "from his mother's womb/Untimely ripped" (5.8.15–16). Disrupted and unnatural motion is thus complicit in the destruction of Macbeth. Critics have noted that the end of the play echoes its beginning: enemies are punished, friends are promised rewards, a head is displayed on a stake. Malcolm attempts to restore a sense of natural teleology and orderly movement: "what's more to do/Which would be planted newly with the time" will be accomplished "in measure, time, and place" (5.9.30–1, 39). However, it seems possible that these measured actions will be perceived by someone as a suffocating blockage, to be followed by another violent purge.

It is hard to imagine how we might evaluate the actual kinesic effects of the images I have been tracing on an audience, or how we would determine whether they are influenced by them for ill (prompted to identify with Macbeth's violent breaching of confining structures) or good (prompted to see that his violent actions ultimately create the conditions for more stringent confinement). The authors of early modern anti-theatrical tracts argued that plays were especially dangerous when they acted on the feelings, rather than the rational understanding, of the audience: "Tragedies and Commedies stirre up affections, and affections are naturally planted in that part of the minde that is common to us with brute beastes."[28] Mary Floyd Wilson has argued that "early modern anti-theatricalists believed that spectators should be concerned about the occult or secret effects of theatre: theatrical performances take 'possession by subtle invasion,' the players' 'impressions of the mind are secretly conveyed to the gazers,' and their 'wanton speeches do pierce our secret thoughts.'"[29] The pre-conscious stage of motor resonance with striking images of physical movement such as the ones I have been tracing in *Macbeth* might well count as a kind of "subtle invasion" that is "secretly conveyed." Even if the imagery of confinement ultimately turns audience sympathy against Macbeth, the unconscious nature of its operation would in itself have been cause for uneasiness.

As I noted at the beginning of this essay, there is, in fact, evidence that readers tend not to be conscious of (or apply conscious analysis to) the pattern of imagery I have been tracing here. In recent articles, both Donald C. Freeman and Howard Marchitello trace an almost unanimous critical reaction to the play, going back to the eighteenth century and extending to the present, that the play conveys a powerful sense of unimpeded forward motion. In Freeman's words "nearly every critic who has written at length on this play has described Macbeth's career as a rushing journey or a series of steps."[30] Similarly, Marchitello notes that "the speed of events in *Macbeth*—and the speed of the play itself—has long been felt."[31] Between them they cite Hazlitt (who describes Macbeth as "blindly rushing forward on the objects of his ambition and revenge"), Coleridge (*Macbeth* is "the most rapid of all Shakespeare's plays"), A. C. Bradley ("our experience in traversing [*Macbeth*] is so crowded and intense that it leaves an impression not of brevity but of speed"), Harry Levin (Macbeth "is the most energetic role in the most intense of Shakespeare's plays") and others as evidence of this near-universal reaction to the play.[32] Some of these readers do notice that there are impediments to Macbeth's rapid forward progress. Freeman quotes Bradley describing how Macbeth "strides from crime to crime, though his soul never ceases to bar his advance with shapes of terror."[33] But in all cases the emphasis is emphatically on Macbeth's intense, energetic and rapid forward motion rather than on conditions, whether internal or external, that would impede him.

Although the older critics do not hesitate to apply moral judgment against Macbeth and his actions, their experience of the play as a successful tragic drama seems dependent upon the speed and intensity of its trajectory. In fact, in Harold Toliver's early moralistic reading of the play, Macbeth's moral failure is represented by his rejection of "measured duration and proper promotion" and his attempt to "escape nature and break the chain of cause and effect" through an ambitious and wilful "trying to overleap time."[34] Toliver assumes that nature is orderly and hierarchical, and tries to claim that the imagery of "stifling" is an effect of Macbeth's ambition rather than its cause. In fact, as I have argued, the play pretty clearly associates stifling, smothering stasis with nature and the political status quo in Scotland even before Macbeth's reign.

Donald Freeman's emphasis on speed in the play is employed in the interest of arguing that the Lakoffian image schemas CONTAINER and PATH shape the play in fundamental ways, with the PATH schema causing its effects of speed: the "unity and focus" of the play in Freeman's argument come from "the almost unbearable intensity with which Shakespeare concentrates our understanding of this play on these two central schemata."[35] Here Freeman writes as if Shakespeare is consciously employing these image schemata in order to create a conscious effect in the audience, although his overall argument is that the play represents "a prototypical case" of the use of image schemata that is "so universal and so central" to human thought and language and presumably acting pre-consciously much of the time.[36] In Freeman's reading, "Macbeth sees the course of our life generally as a potentially obstacle-laden journey along a path or way," a view that seems to reflect some level of identification with Macbeth, even though the CONTAINER schema throws up barriers in the way of the PATH, which ultimately leads to nothing.[37] The PATH schema itself, however, does tend to put a positive valence on forward movement and agency, imagining obstacles as there to be overcome. Freeman's reading may therefore show how a conscious perception of (and investment in) headlong rush can be primed by a pre-conscious perception of an atmosphere replete with impediments.

Marchitello is up to something quite different, using the French cultural theorist Paul Virilio and his theories about speed to understand the trajectory of the play. For Marchitello "Macbeth's violent and frenetic actions are less the consequences of a certain pathology and more the manifestation of what it means to exist in a world radically accelerated toward a mode of being (Virilio would say a 'milieu') in which temporality collapses into functional instantaneity."[38] Marchitello argues that the witches represent an intervention of supernatural "absolute speed," which "engenders and determines Macbeth's will to power, however self-defeating it proves to be."[39] Speed is here imagined as a cultural rather than moral or psychological phenomenon, but it is still regarded with rapt fascination, while images of thick, suffocating impediment do not seem to register. Marchitello, for instance, misses the fact that the witches' first effect is to bring Macbeth to an abrupt stop, and does not comment on the many images of choking, strangling and sticking to be found in the play. The evidence that Marchitello finds to support his contention that the play is characterized by speed depends less on kinesic images than on the play's brevity and on its references to time. Marchitello cites A. C. Bradley and Harry Levin who link the play's effects of speed to its status as Shakespeare's shortest play, and Stephen Orgel who blames its temporal disruptions on the uncertain state of the text.[40] Although Marchitello argues that "speed and its effects can be felt beyond what seem to be obvious or apparent cuts and revisions" (431), most of the evidence for this felt effect of speed lies in statements expressing the Macbeths' "impatience with temporality" (447). I would argue that the play lets us feel the reasons for Macbeth's impatience more powerfully and kinetically than it expresses his speed.

While analysis of the imagery of speed in the play is strongly associated with moral judgment of the Macbeths (and the witches), the speed critics nevertheless seem fascinated by and even swept up in Macbeth's "headlong rush" toward his ultimate fate. It does seem possible that a preconscious experience of stifling, strangling, impediment contributes to what seems almost to be a state of exhilaration in its effects of speed, which is then managed by explicit condemnation of Macbeth's ambitious violation of natural order. Of course, a play that depicted characters who were stuck, whose movements were persistently thwarted, who did not speed toward a purposeful goal, would be quite a different play: *Hamlet*, perhaps, or more literally Samuel Beckett's *Happy Days* where the main character is buried up to her waist and then, in act 2, up to her neck and cannot move at all. It makes sense that readers like the critics cited above respond to the intensity of *Macbeth*, resonating with the desperate and frantic efforts of Macbeth to attain, and then hold onto, the Scottish throne. It does seem possible, however, that this response is unconsciously primed by the sense of confinement and frustration that makes Macbeth's rash actions seem so compelling. Shakespeare need not have intended the double kinesic effect of this play. Any text—even, as we saw, Cleanth Brooks's essay on *Macbeth*—will reflect the embodied origins of language through imagery that naturally expresses the ways in which human feeling is bound up with bodily posture and movement. And it is not only drama that conveys hidden "impressions of the mind" through a "subtle invasion," as early modern anti-theatricalists feared. All language, especially densely metaphoric literary language, strikes the reader, and causes resonances, that we do not necessarily perceive consciously. Attention to kinesis represents a way to bring some of these hidden resonances to light.

Interestingly, two of the early "speed" critics, Harold Toliver and Donald Foster, recognize a fundamental "paradox" or "irony" in the play.[41] In Toliver's words, "the central paradox of the play is that the most depraved of Shakespeare's tragic heroes should have become also its most 'poetic,'" noting that Macbeth's language is "illuminating and rich beyond that of other Shakespearean tragic heroes."[42] "Paradox" brings us back to Cleanth Brooks, and his contention that the task of literary analysis is to identify in imagery, which may or may not be consciously intended, the foundational paradoxes that characterize poetic language. It seems likely to me that the powerful kinesic images of smothering and stasis that these critics more or less ignore in their conscious analysis are what provide some of their sense that the play is uniquely "poetic." Although it is impossible to know how pre-conscious motor resonance has influenced readings that do not attend to it, it seems possible that the relationship between pre-conscious experience of these images and intentional analysis of the imagery of the play is not continuous or straightforward. Attention to kinesis may help us to understand more fully the force of poetic language in ways that we have not previously been able to notice.

Notes

1. W. K. Wimsatt and M. C. Beardsley, "The Intentional Fallacy," *The Sewanee Review* 54 (1946): 468. See also Cleanth Brooks, in *The Well Wrought Urn: Studies in the Structure of Poetry* (New York: Harvest, 1947), 22–49 ("The Naked Babe and the Cloak of Manliness").
2. Brooks, 23.

3. Brooks, 3–4.
4. Brooks, 48.
5. Brooks, 24.
6. Brooks, 26.
7. Brooks, 45–6, 49, 48.
8. Introduction, p. 0000.
9. Terence Cave, *Thinking with Literature: Towards a Cognitive Criticism* (Oxford: Oxford University Press, 2016), 23.
10. Harold E. Toliver, "Shakespeare and the Abyss of Time," *JEGP* 64, no. 2 (1965): 248.
11. Toliver, 247.
12. See Toliver, also Donald W. Foster, "Macbeth's War on Time," *ELR* 16, no. 2 (1986): 319–342 as well as Howard Marchitello, "Speed and the Problem of Real Time in *Macbeth*," *Shakespeare Quarterly* 64, no. 4 (Winter 2013): 425–448.
13. Stephen Greenblatt, "Shakespeare Bewitched," in *Shakespeare and Cultural Traditions*, ed. Tetsuo Kishi, Roger Pringle, and Stanley Wells (Newark: University of Delaware Press, 1994), 17–42. See also Peter Stallybrass, "*Macbeth* and Witchcraft," in *Focus on Macbeth*, ed. John Russell Brown, (London: Routledge and Kegan Paul, 1982), 189–209 and Janet Adelman, "'Born of Woman': Fantasies of Maternal Power in *Macbeth*," in *Cannibals, Witches, and Divorce: Estranging the Renaissance*, ed. Marjorie Garber (Baltimore: Johns Hopkins University Press, 1987), 90–121.
14. For example, see Amy Cook, *Shakespearean Neuroplay: Reinvigorating the Study of Dramatic Texts and Performance through Cognitive Science* (New York: Palgrave, 2010); and Naomi Rokotnitz, "'It is required/You do awake your faith': Learning to trust the body through performing *The Winter's Tale*," in *Performance and Cognition: Theatre Studies and the Cognitive Turn*, ed. Bruce McConachie and F. Elizabeth Hart (New York: Routledge, 2006), 122–146.
15. As I will discuss at the end of this essay, other critics have noticed images of obstacles in the play. They have tended not to link obstacles with images of atmospheric and humoral thickness and choking, however.
16. Stuart Clark, *Vanities of the Eye: Vision in Early Modern European Culture* (Oxford: Oxford University Press, 2007), 236–265.
17. Werner Habicht, "'And Mock Our Eyes with Air': Air and Stage Illusion in Shakespearean Drama," in *Aesthetic Illusion*, ed. Frederick Burwick and Walter Pape (Berlin: de Gruyter, 1990), 301–312.
18. Mary Floyd-Wilson, "English Epicures and Scottish Witches," *Shakespeare Quarterly* 57 (2006): 131–161.
19. See, for example, Brooks.
20. Clark, 248.

21. G. Blakemore Evans, ed., *The Riverside Shakespeare* (Boston: Houghton Mifflin, 1974). All citations from *Macbeth* are from this edition.
22. Marchitello associates the witches with speed because they can appear and disappear instantaneously. But he doesn't take into account the images of thick air and "starting" that arrest as well as impel motion.
23. Floyd-Wilson notes that Scottish sources associate witches with an ability to control the wind; "English Epicures," 148.
24. See Guillemette Bolens, *The Style of Gestures: Embodiment and Cognition in Literary Narrative* (Baltimore: Johns Hopkins University Press, 2012), 29–31, for the discussion of the kinesic impact of "starting" that Banks and Chesters mention in the introduction to this volume. Bolens notes that Darcy's start is in itself a strong kinesic reaction" which also induces "the complex perceptual simulation of a contained and constrained yet briefly overwhelming general movement" (29–30). She emphasizes the cultural context for Darcy's containment and constraint. Macbeth's start and raptness occur in a different context and represent a different, but no less striking, form of constraint.
25. Shakespeare uses the word "rapt" only seven times in his plays, three of which occur in the first act of *Macbeth.*
26. Janet Adelman, *Suffocating Mothers: Fantasies of Maternal Origin in Shakespeare's Plays, Hamlet to the Tempest* (New York: Routledge, 1992), 135.
27. Donald C. Freeman discusses many of the metaphors that I note here; see his "'Catch[ing] the nearest way': *Macbeth* and Cognitive Metaphor," *Journal of Pragmatics* 24 (1995): 689–708. He explains them as manifestations of Lakoff and Johnson's PATH image schema. I discuss his reading in more detail at the end of this essay.
28. Stephen Gosson, "Playes Confuted in five Actions" (1582), cited in *The Elizabethan Stage*, ed. E. K. Chambers, (Oxford: Clarendon, 1923), 4: 217.
29. Mary Floyd Wilson, *Occult Knowledge, Science, and Gender on the Shakespearean Stage* (Cambridge: Cambridge University Press, 2013), 21. Floyd Wilson is citing William Rankins, "A Mirror of Monsters" (1587), Stephen Gosson, "Plays Confuted in Five Actions" (1582), Anthony Munday, "A Second and Third Blast of Retreat from Plays and Theater (1580) as taken from *Shakespeare's Theater: A Sourcebook*, ed. Tanya Pollard (Oxford: Blackwell, 2004), 125, 108, 79.
30. Freeman, 689.
31. Marchitello, 430.
32. Freeman cites William Hazlitt from *The Characters of Shakespeare's Plays*, ed. Arthur Quiller Couch (Oxford: Oxford University Press, 1939), 14; "Catch[ing] the nearest way," 690. Marchitello cites Coleridge from

Samuel Taylor Coleridge, *The Literary Remains of Samuel Taylor Coleridge*, ed. Henry Nelson Coleridge, (London: Pickering, 1836–1839), 2:235; A. C. Bradley, *Shakespearean Tragedy: Lectures on "Hamlet," "Othello," "King Lear," "Macbeth,"* (London: Macmillan, 1904), 333; Harry Levin, "Two Scenes from *Macbeth*" in *Shakespeare's Craft: Eight Lectures*, ed. Philip H. Highfill Jr. (Carbondale, Southern Illinois UP, 1982), 48.

33. Freeman cites the same edition of Bradley's *Shakespearean Tragedy*; "Catch[ing] the nearest way," 361.
34. Toliver, 247.
35. Freeman, 693.
36. Freeman, 691, 707.
37. Freeman, 702.
38. Marchitello, 433.
39. Marchitello, 444.
40. Marchitello, 430–1.
41. Toliver, 250; Foster, 337.
42. Toliver, 250.

Bibliography

Adelman, Janet. 'Born of Woman': Fantasies of Maternal Power in *Macbeth*. In *Cannibals, Witches, and Divorce: Estranging the Renaissance*, edited by Marjorie Garber, 90–121. Baltimore: Johns Hopkins University Press, 1987.

———. *Suffocating Mothers: Fantasies of Maternal Origin in Shakespeare's Plays, Hamlet to the Tempest*. New York: Routledge, 1992.

Blakemore Evans, Gwynne, ed. *The Riverside Shakespeare*. Boston: Houghton Mifflin, 1974.

Bolens, Guillemette. *The Style of Gestures: Embodiment and Cognition in Literary Narrative*. Baltimore: Johns Hopkins University Press, 2012.

Bradley, A. C. *Shakespearean Tragedy: Lectures on "Hamlet," "Othello," "King Lear," "Macbeth."* London: Macmillan, 1904.

Brooks, Cleanth. *The Well Wrought Urn: Studies in the Structure of Poetry*. New York: Harvest, 1947; rpt. 1975.

Cave, Terence. *Thinking with Literature: Towards a Cognitive Criticism*. Oxford: Oxford University Press, 2016.

Chambers, E. K., ed. *The Elizabethan Stage*. Vol. 4. Oxford: Clarendon, 1923.

Clark, Stuart. *Vanities of the Eye: Vision in Early Modern European Culture*. Oxford: Oxford University Press, 2007.

Coleridge, Samuel Taylor. *The Literary Remains of Samuel Taylor Coleridge*, edited by Henry Nelson Coleridge. 4 vols. London: Pickering, 1836–1839.

Cook, Amy. *Shakespearean Neuroplay: Reinvigorating the Study of Dramatic Texts and Performance Through Cognitive Science*. New York: Palgrave, 2010.

Floyd-Wilson, Mary. English Epicures and Scottish Witches. *Shakespeare Quarterly* 57 (2006): 131–161.

———. *Occult Knowledge, Science, and Gender on the Shakespearean Stage.* Cambridge: Cambridge University Press, 2013.

Foster, Donald W. Macbeth's War on Time. *ELR* 16, no. 2 (1986): 319–342.

Freeman, Donald C. 'Catch[ing] the nearest way': *Macbeth* and Cognitive Metaphor. *Journal of Pragmatics* 24 (1995): 689–708.

Greenblatt, Stephen. Shakespeare Bewitched. In *Shakespeare and Cultural Traditions*, edited by Tetsuo Kishi, Roger Pringle, and Stanley Wells, 17–42. Newark: University of Delaware Press, 1994.

Habicht, Werner. 'And Mock Our Eyes with Air': Air and Stage Illusion in Shakespearean Drama. In *Aesthetic Illusion*, edited by Frederick Burwick and Walter Pape, 301–312. Berlin: de Gruyter, 1990.

Levin, Harry. Two Scenes from Macbeth. In *Shakespeare's Craft: Eight Lectures*, edited by Philip H. Highfill Jr. Carbondale: Southern Illinois UP, 1982.

Marchitello, Howard. Speed and the Problem of Real Time in Macbeth. *Shakespeare Quarterly* 64, no. 4 (Winter 2013): 425–448.

Pollard, Tanya, ed. *Shakespeare's Theater: A Sourcebook.* Oxford: Blackwell, 2004.

Quiller Couch, Arthur, ed. *The Characters of Shakespeare's Plays.* Oxford: Oxford University Press, 1939.

Rokotnitz, Naomi. 'It Is Required/You do Awake Your Faith': Learning to Trust the Body Through Performing *The Winter's Tale.* In *Performance and Cognition: Theatre Studies and the Cognitive Turn*, edited by Bruce McConachie and F. Elizabeth Hart, 122–146. New York: Routledge, 2006.

Stallybrass, Peter. *Macbeth* and Witchcraft. In *Focus on Macbeth*, edited by John Russell Brown, 189–209. London: Routledge and Kegan Paul, 1982.

Toliver, Harold E. Shakespeare and the Abyss of Time. *JEGP* 64, no. 2 (1965): 234–254.

Wimsatt, W. K., and M. C. Beardsley. The Intentional Fallacy. *The Sewanee Review* 54, no. 3 (1946): 468–488.

CHAPTER 10

Shakespeare's Vital Signs

Raphael Lyne

When our son was nine years old we went to see the film *Avatar* (2009). He was overwhelmed by the 3D CGI extravaganza, and at one point he began to worry that he might, in his excitement, have stopped breathing. In the cinema, we were unable to convince him that he was alright, and it took a little walk in the calm foyer to reacquaint him with the routine, usually unconscious, sensations of respiration. His tenacity in refusing to acknowledge that he must be breathing, or that he could access evidence of his breathing by deliberately drawing in and expelling air, was striking. It can be hard to prove, especially to yourself, that you are, in the simplest sense, alive, and have not unwittingly ebbed away because the world has proved too intense or diverting. These signs may resist or reward careful attention in life, and in the theatre too. Shakespeare takes a keen interest in these proofs and tests in a striking number of plays. They are, it turns out, a special case of the kind of "kinesic intelligence" that is at issue throughout this volume. The actor's performance of just being alive makes us think about the boundary between animation and its opposite; it exposes aspects of the process of drama itself, bringing unnoticed things to light; and it reflects back on our sensorimotor capacities in their rawness and their virtuosity.

R. Lyne (✉)
Murray Edwards College, Cambridge, UK

K. Banks, T. Chesters (eds.), *Movement in Renaissance Literature*, Cognitive Studies in Literature and Performance,
https://doi.org/10.1007/978-3-319-69200-5_10

***

In one of Shakespeare's earliest plays, King Henry VI struggles to face up to the fickleness of his fortunes and his people. One says that they were his true sworn subjects, "while you were king," at which he protests:

> Why? Am I dead? Do I not breathe a man?
> Ah, simple men, you know not what you swear!
> Look, as I blow this feather from my face,
> And as the air blows it to me again,
> Obeying with my wind when I do blow,
> And yielding to another when it blows,
> Commanded always by the greater gust,
> Such is the lightness of you common men. (3.1.82–9)[1]

The feather is a symbol of the changeability of popular opinion, always victim to "the greater gust." However, it also performs another role, proving that Henry is still breathing, still alive, and thus, in his view, the King. There is a similar role for a feather in *Henry IV Part II*, though in that case it provides a false indication of death. Prince Hal is left alone with his ailing father, and becomes convinced that his father is no longer breathing:

> By his gates of breath
> There lies a downy feather which stirs not.
> Did he suspire, that light and weightless down
> Perforce must move. My gracious lord! My father!
> This sleep is sound indeed, this is a sleep
> That from this golden rigol hath divorc'd
> So many English kings. (4.5.31–7)

The prince takes up the golden "rigol," the crown, an object that has exerted so much pressure on his father, but which also represents his own destiny. The feather seems to be a different kind of theatrical object from the one in *Henry VI Part 3*. This is the kind of tiny white feather that might happen to appear on a King's face as he lies in bed, just part of the bedding itself, and probably invisible to the audience. The one blown by the King in his subjects' faces would probably be visible, a stage prop, rather than an imaginary thing, although the movements it is asked to make are rather precise.[2]

Soon after this, the King wakes up, calling for "Warwick! Gloucester! Clarence!," finding himself without a crown (48). This leads to painful confrontation with Hal: "Is he so hasty that he doth suppose / My sleep my death?" (60–1). But who, in that moment, did not? In the end the two are reconciled, when the Prince convinces his father that he was full of grief. In between two peaks of emotional intensity (Hal believing himself to be King; the reconciliation of father and son) there is a moment with a special sort of dramatic intensity. An actor has to establish that the character he is playing is alive. There is no stage direction, and no readily available type of stage of direction in Shakespeare's time, to convey *He Is Alive*. Presumably, however, the moment before the King speaks covers a moment in which his vital signs become evident again: a sudden stir, a gasp of breath, opening eyes, an indication of awareness. Between the *Exit* of Hal and the *Enter* of "Warwick, Gloucester, Clarence, [*and the rest*]," as the Riverside puts it, the only thing in the text is the King crying out the three names. This could, perhaps must be, a slow moment on stage nonetheless, where the audience waits for something to happen, and what happens is life.

These two instances, emphatic and then misleading uses of breath-revealing feathers, are part of Shakespeare's career-long interest in the basic signs of life. Repeatedly he comes back to breath, movement, pulse, warmth, a sense of weight borne rather than slumping, those things that indicate life-rather-than-death. This interest is partly a matter of plot, and the various tensions and thrills that are associated with the figure who might be dead, or who is thought to be dead. It is partly, and crucially, a matter of performance: life itself is part of the actor's art, and it is a test and demonstration of that art to isolate *life alone* as something to be acted. As has already been seen, these moments of uncertainty enable strange things to happen to stage time. How long the king should wait, and how sudden or dramatic his revival should be, are questions left dynamically open.

This is both a foundational and a special case of kinesic intelligence at work. It is atypical, in that lacks a meaningful gesture or a purposeful action. The paradigmatic instances described in the Introduction to this volume involve embodied responses to movements described or hinted at, from which may or must be inferred significant intentions or feelings. When it comes to the vital signs of Shakespearean characters, what is inferred is just *life*, up to a point. Guillemette Bolens, however, anticipates this possibility by referring to literature's capacity to evoke the complexity of the kinesic world. Recognizing the sensorimotor component in literary response does not always clarify the workings of a text; sometimes a writer may be testing out that very component, extending our understanding of its processes. So, as Bolens says, "Proust shows what is at stake in kinesic expression, warding off, through the style of his prose and the force of his description, the temptation to limit or simplify our sense of human expressiveness"; and more generally, "art creates obstacles to the oversimplification of human expression."[3]

Terence Cave has pointed out that the ability to recognize living things is a crucial function of human cognition. Of all the things in the environment being surveyed by our senses, these are the greatest threats and opportunities. And yet, as he says, "recognition of life, despite its cognitive complexity, comes too naturally for us to be able to analyse it."[4] Cave also emphasizes the "assumption of *agency*… a peculiar kind of directedness… an intention which may be more or less overt." In so many cases, of course, this agency is overwhelmingly important, but in the dramatic moments featured in this essay, the identification of life may briefly lack an impression of intentionality, at least on the part of the character. The agency of the actor comes into special focus, and the ability to analyse this is more easily exercised.

Our responses to characters on the boundary between life and death, then, may enable possible rediscovery of the sensations of vitality, and they may also highlight the strangeness of the things on which we utterly depend. Even though the consequences of *not-death* are usually enormous, the thing that is simulated, thought through with the body, may at times be isolated as mere animation, the sensations of being sentient and functioning even before the context begins to impinge. Perhaps the enormity of what awaits the waker cannot entirely be set aside. However, this is where the emergence of the actor as the focus of kinesic intelligence makes a special difference. The theatre has proved fertile territory for cognitive approaches not least because they have offered new ways of thinking about the "conceptual blend" of actor and character.[5] It seems intuitively right, as well as theoretically sound, to assume that kinesic intelligence attends to both, and perhaps to various kinds of merger. So the theatre is a special location for thinking through such responses, and in this case it is particularly suggestive to think about how the skill of acting vital signs may be isolated. One route to a fuller understanding of what it is to be alive is to think about what it would take to pretend not to be, and then to be (or vice versa).

***

The paradigmatic case, as far as criticism is concerned, is the coming-to-life of the statue of Hermione in *The Winter's Tale*. Here there is a particular complexity to the craft of acting involved. The statue is a pretend statue: in the end it is apparent that the Queen has been kept alive in the hope that things will turn out well. The statue deception helps produce the right posture of submissive compliance in Leontes, her husband. However, the way in which the actor pretends to be a statue as it stands on a pedestal, and the way in which the character is pretending, are not the same thing. There is something mysterious about Hermione's preservation, and it doesn't seem right to think of this as an act; meanwhile the actor has to play the part of a different human being not quite playing at being a work of art.

These multiple mediations frame, without diluting, the coming-to-life experience that the audience shares, hyper-aware of those initial movements, the warmth and breath and the experience of warmth and breath, all of which are afforded careful attention in Shakespeare. Some of this, as will be seen, is disarmingly explicit, while some (like the moment of Henry IV's revival) is manifest only in the space left for it to appear. Hannah Chapelle Wojciehowski has illuminated the "vitality effects" of the scene.[6] Inspired by research into embodied simulation and mirroring, and by many of the key reference points for the study of "kinesic intelligence," she argues for the audience's intimate acquaintance with these vital signs: "As we watch the 'statue' stir (however that stirring may be performed), we *become* Hermione for a moment. Her return to vitality (or rather, the actress's or actor's performance thereof) is mirrored within us alteroceptively; it ripples through our bodies."[7]

Wojciehowski turns towards Ellen Spolsky's work on the "cognitive hunger" of post-Reformation England.[8] She sees the final scene of *The Winter's Tale* as a staging of the residual energy of Catholic visual art: the energy of these palpable representations of feeling was still felt. For the concept of vitality Wojciehowski looks to Daniel Stern's exploration of "dynamic experience."[9] In Stern's work, vitality is a "Gestalt" made up of "movement, time, force, space and intention/directionality" (pp. 4–5). He is interested in the "experience of vitality" at the minimal level represented in Shakespeare, but it usually seems to be a prelude to greater leaps and bends, something constantly with us: "if our breath and body were not in a constant process of change when awake, we would not feel alive and vital" (p. 9). Citing Merleau-Ponty's *Phenomenology of Perception* on the phenomenological idea of "the upsurge of a fresh present" Stern is focused on "arousal systems," the alertness and in-the-momentness of experience.[10]

This idea of vitality might be compared and contrasted with the one in Garrett Sullivan's recent book on the fortunes of the Aristotelian tripartite soul in renaissance literature.[11] For Aristotle, the soul consisted of three parts: the vegetative (associated with plants), sensitive (associated with animals) and rational (associated only with humans). Sullivan argues that understanding vitality at key moments in Renaissance literature requires an understanding of this tripartite quality. The legacy of Descartes, Sullivan argues, was to take out everything but the rational soul from what characterized the human. The philosophical cost implied here overlaps with that identified in Antonio Damasio's *Descartes' Error*, which set itself up as an attempt to reacquaint mind and body.[12] The literary-critical cost, for Sullivan, is a failure to understand that the soul is at issue when, for example, physical sensitivity is evoked. In Spenser and even in Milton the fullness of Aristotelian vitality is often to be seen.

Sullivan is interested in sleep as a plot motif where the definition of the vital soul comes into view. Like Stern, however, he is not interested in the details of the boundary between vitality and its opposite. Despite the excellent work of Wojciehowski and others on the *The Winter's Tale* scene, there is still more to notice in its meticulous attention to signs of life.[13] Paulina urges Leontes to give his own meticulous attention to the statue by inviting him to compare it with his memory of his wife: "comes it not something near?" (5.3.23). Soon afterwards, however, she begins to withdraw the offer:

PAULINA No longer shall you gaze on't, lest your fancy
May think anon it moves.
LEONTES Let be, let be.
Would I were dead but that, methinks, already—
What was he that did make it? See, my lord,
Would you not deem it breath'd? and that those veins
Did verily bear blood?
POLIXENES Masterly done!
The very life seems warm upon her lip.
LEONTES The fixure of her eye has motion in't,
As we are mock'd with art.
PAULINA I'll draw the curtain.
My lord's almost so far transported that
He'll think anon it lives. (5.3.60–70)

In this exchange some of the key vital signs, which will run throughout the scene, are listed: motion, breath, pulse, warmth, and some sort of presence in the eye—someone at home. A dazzling twist of plot, the chance for some virtuosic acting (is the point to represent the absence of these things, their covert presence, their potential?), and the burden on the cooperative audience (what are we supposed to see here, and what are we supposed to look for?), are all combined. "We are mock'd with art" applies to the audience as well as to the characters, and to acting as well as sculpture. This is very purposeful and productive meta-theatrical play, though: it heightens the already unbearable scrutiny that is being loaded onto this scene, reaching in several different under-focused ways after tell-tale hints.

When the statue finally comes to life, the emphasis is mostly on movement. Paulina calls for music and then addresses the statue:

> 'Tis time; descend; be stone no more; approach;
> Strike all that look upon with marvel. Come;
> I'll fill your grave up. Stir; nay, come away;
> Bequeath to death your numbness; for from him
> Dear life redeems you. You perceive she stirs. (5.3.99–103)

There is a difference between "stir" (the barest sign of animation in motion) and "descend"; the latter, though a more purposeful and directed movement, denotes another quality of liveliness. The actor playing Hermione, if being stone, must not project the sensation of weight. To "descend" is to encounter gravity directly, to move with it and let it direct the body. It is no coincidence, then, that after another iconic encounter with vitality (Leontes: "O, she's warm!") the observers describe another gravity-oriented interaction:

> POLIXENES She embraces him.
> CAMILLO She hangs about his neck:
> If she pertain to life let her speak too. (5.3.111–13)

Camillo has his eye in the end on another clinching sign of life: speech would make this a person, not a charmed artwork. The entry into language might denote the end of this particular moment of kinesic attunement to vital signs: there is something fuller, less particular, less obscure in the actor's art, when it takes the form of words. Before making that turn he offers an elaboration of Polixenes' description that conveys the intensity of the embrace but also its sense of weight. Hermione shares that sign of life:

a body has to support itself or be supported, and posture (tension and/or relaxation, rather than stony stillness) is one of Shakespeare's vital signs.

Although this scene has been discussed many times, without all of these kinesic possibilities having been recognized as such, its significance in relation to vitality truly is enhanced by comparison with the many other moments in Shakespeare where life is in question. Audiences are made to consider their own attentiveness (are we looking to see if the actor is breathing, or not?) and also their own sense of what being alive is like. It is difficult to imagine what it would be like to have no breath, but what these plays encourage us to simulate is not just what it would be like to find breath when there was none, but also what it would take to perform that arrival into breath (and warmth, pulse, weight, stirring, etc.). The actor is a tangible means of reaching something intangible: by reconceiving life as a matter of technique we estrange ourselves from qualities that may only be tangible because of that estrangement.

***

The romances written around the same time as *The Tempest* share an interest in the return to life. Though the methods and circumstances are different, the moments of tension in simulation and performance are similar. In *Pericles* Thaisa is buried at sea after dying in childbirth, but her coffin washes up on a shore where there happens to be someone with superior medical-magical skill. Cerimon says that "Death may usurp on nature many hours, / And yet the fire of life kindle again / The o'erpress'd spirits" (3.2.82–4). He traces the signs of that rekindling, and the audience must observe the details of the actor passing through explicit stages: "Nature awakes, / A warmth breathes out of her… See how she gins / To blow into life's flower again!" (3.2.92–5). The mixture of metaphor here gets at the problem of comprehension and performance: Nature (not she) awakes; warmth is felt in the form of a breath that may or may not be an expulsion or inhalation; the "blow" hints at breath and movement but takes the form of a figurative flower. Smell has already been a feature of the scene, though an unreachable one for the audience: the body is notably "fresh" (79), which is what sets Cerimon thinking in the first place.

He goes on to describe something that surely must be a cue for the actor, something explicit and specific that makes the earlier life-signs seem all the more tenuous:

She is alive; behold
Her eyelids, cases to those heavenly jewels
Which Pericles hath lost, begin to part
Their fringes of bright gold. The diamonds
Of a most praised water doth appear,
To make the world twice rich. Live, and make
Us weep to hear your fate, fair creature,
Rare as you seem to be. (3.2.97–104)

Paulina asks the statue to re-enter the world, and here Cerimon does the same. His cue is the opening of her eyes and the appearance of a tear. Alongside any application of kinesic intelligence to the experience of the character here, there is a more achievable one to the practice of the actor, blinking as moistly as possible as a prelude to a set of believable questions: "Where am I? Where's my lord? What world is this?" This time there is a stage direction (in the earliest edition, the Quarto of 1609; *Pericles* is not in the first Folio), directly after the speech above and before she speaks: *She moves.*

When, in *Cymbeline*, Imogen wakes from her drugged and death-like sleep (death-like enough that she has been mourned), she also has questions.[14] This time they are poised between some kind of dream-state, in which she is still searching for Posthumus, and the immediate reality:

Yes, sir, to Milford-Haven, which is the way?
I thank you. By yond bush? Pray how far thither?
'Ods pittikins! can it be six mile yet?
I have gone all night. 'Faith, I'll lie down and sleep. (4.2.291–4)

What is distinctive here is the portrayal of cognitive awakening, the difficulty of composing lucid thoughts at such a moment. Imogen is noticeably less poised than Hermione and Thaisa. There is nothing specific in the Folio text to guide the actor before the speech beyond a direction "*Imogen awakes*" after the "*Exeunt*" of the mourners. Again the durations of the gap before the waking, the waking process, and the gap between waking and speech, are left open. Here too there has to be some sort of return to vitality: something intensely watched, of indeterminate length, characterized by familiar signs, which marks the transition from a state that could convince people of death, into one that is ready for speech.

Shakespeare replays the process by having Imogen faint, as if dead, when she thinks that the headless body beside her is that of Posthumus. When the Roman army enters, then, she is taken for dead for a second time.

> How? a page?
> Or dead, or sleeping on him? But dead rather;
> For nature doth abhor to make his bed
> With the defunct, or sleep upon the dead.
> Let's see the boy's face. (4.2.355–9)

Lucius's reasons for thinking that Imogen is dead are superficial, and on what might be very brief closer inspection a Captain discovers that she is actually alive. This is still a kind of rebirth, even if it requires a bit less tension and technique around the signs of life. Imogen says at first "I am nothing," eventually claiming a new name, "Fidele." So Shakespeare has produced a two-stage encounter with the problem and opportunity of coming to life.

The second awakening replays the first; and Imogen also replays, here, the awakening of Thaisa, and perhaps most of all the awakening of Juliet (which will be discussed below). Hermione's statue is a development and revisiting of Thaisa and Imogen, and of Juliet perhaps, but most of all of Cleopatra (who will also be discussed below). These are only the Shakespearean inter-references. Other versions of the revival story, or the transition from an inanimate to an animate state (as in the Pygmalion story, well known to Shakespeare's time in Ovid's and other versions), are also being revisited here.[15] The intensity of attention results partly from the many variations on the signs of liveliness in literary and dramatic tradition.

***

It also arises from a particular set of ideas and questions about this boundary that pertained in Shakespearean England. In writings about life and death, not surprisingly, the phenomena involved are often approached from the other side: vital signs are switched off rather than on. They can, in some physiological contexts, be reversible. Kaara Peterson has written about the affinity between Shakespeare's various representations of reviving women, and the symptoms of the hysteria-related disorder "the

Suffocation of the Mother."[16] This could produce symptoms akin to death, and it could result in sudden revival. Peterson cites Edward Jorden's description of the disease from 1603. The way he traces the decline of the "vital function" of the heart does display an acute interest in the signs of life alluded to in the plays. In some cases the pulse "is oftentimes diminished either in part or to sense totally":

> It is totally diminished in that Symptom which is called Syncope or swounding, the very image of death, where the pulse is scarcely or not at all perceyved; the breath or respiration cleane gone: by reason that the heart wanting his motion, hath no neede of the helpe of the lungs to refresh it withall, all the faculties of the body fayling, it self lying like a dead corpse three or foure houres togither, and sometimes two or three whole dayes without sense, motion, breath, heate, or any signe of life at all (like as wee see Snakes and other creatures to lie all the winter, as if they were dead, under the earth) insomuch as diverse errors have beene committed in laying foorth such for dead, which have afterwards beene found to have life in them, and have risen up in their burials.[17]

Anecdotes that follow describe near-misses and legislative responses to cases where a woman has been nearly buried, or vivisected, as a result of this false appearance of death. Thaisa's situation bears the closest resemblance to the scenario described here, but even the other cases cited thus far, and to follow, are united crucially by gender: female vitality is perhaps especially mysterious, capable of confounding the usual categories.

The boundary of vitality is encountered not just through disease, but also through acts of mind, some more deliberate than others. Typically Montaigne is an acute observer of the strangeness of the human condition. He offers instances—again anecdote is a key resource for the writer—where the power of the imagination has dulled the vital signs to the point of invisibility:

> Othersome will say, that by the force of it, bodies are sometimes removed from their places. And Celsus reportes of a priest, whose soule was ravished into such an extasie, that for a long time the body remained voyde of all exspiration and sence. Saint Augustine speaketh of an other, who if hee but heard any lamentable and wailefull cries, would sodainely fall into a sowne, and bee so forcibly carried from himselfe, that did any chide and braule never so loude, pinch and thumpe him never so much, he could not be made to stirre, untill hee came to himselfe againe. Then would he say, he

> had heard sundry strange voyces, comming as it were from a farre, and perceiving his pinches and bruses, wondered at them. And that it was not an obstinate conceit, or wilfull humour in him, or against his feeling sence, it plainely appeared by this, because during his extasie, he seemed to have neither pulse nor breath.[18]

This is still an ailment of sorts, rather than a skill: none of the cases cited here is using this power of the imagination advisedly. The power of the traumatized mind may somewhat be in evidence in the Shakespearean examples cited so far (especially Imogen) but there are usually plainer causes at stake.

In addition to these two encounters with the ebbing away of vital signs (again it should be emphasized that this is usually the opposite direction from the one represented in Shakespeare's plays), one more context should be adduced. This is the art of dying well, in which the transition out of vitality is one of the things to be managed carefully.

> The disposition of him that dyeth is to be consydered, & to behold the present howre of the separation of the soule from ye fleshe, whereof man hath a naturall feare, for then man altogeather waxeth pale, his feete waxeth colde, his weake hands becommeth blacke, his countenaunce chaungeth colour, his eyes becommeth dimme, and sinketh in, and for intollerable pangues of paynes they are turned upwarde. See how his hart waxeth faynt, his forehead shrinketh, all his members waxeth styffe, his chinne falleth, his pulses chaungeth theyr course, & his breath gathering it self from the innermost bowels doo altogether forsake the body. The paines of death do then appeare, & deadly pangues, stinging with the mortal stinges the very harte, which fyrst of al begynneth to lyve, and last of al doth dye. And last of al there commeth & breaketh foorth a dead sweate, shewing that Nature is overcome. And thus being vanquished by griefe the soule is cast out from hir dwelling place. If we wyl consyder this disposition of them that dye, and do dilygentlie imagine, that the lyke wyl shortlie happen unto our selves, there is no doubte but we wyll consider the healthfull feare of death.[19]

Being prepared for death means understanding its various stages. This way round, the emphasis is on pain and loss, aspects of the process that can be prepared for. Contemplation of the symptoms of life as they disappear (colour, warmth, pulse, breath) is part of preparing for a dignified demeanour as one comes closer to the Almighty. Peterson is surely right to draw attention to 'the Suffocation of the Mother' as an uncannily apt parallel for some aspects of Shakespeare's treatment of vital signs (for example, the connection with sexuality, childbirth, or virginity). Nevertheless it is clear that there are other contexts in which the manifestations of the life-death boundary are of great interest to early modern culture, and this must have helped fuel Shakespeare's repeated returns to the motif.

***

Shakespeare's most memorable instance of the performance of prepared death is Cleopatra. Whereas in *The Winter's Tale* a statue becomes a Queen, here a Queen becomes a statue. Cleopatra has practised, we are told, her own kind of *ars moriendi*, fixing on the asp as a way of dying peacefully. Where De Soto dwells with relish on pain, Cleopatra has pursued an easier way. The actors in the scene (for there are three deaths) are given the challenge of acting out the experience of life being extinguished. First Iras dies:

> Come then, and take the last warmth of my lips.
> Farewell, kind Charmian, Iras, long farewell.
> [*Kisses them. Iras falls and dies.*]
> Have I the aspic in my lips? Dost fall?
> If thou and nature can so gently part,
> The stroke of death is as a lover's pinch,
> Which hurts, and is desir'd. (5.2.291–6)

Cleopatra is depicting her own de-vitalization, sharing her "last warmth," but Iras suddenly succumbs, either to her own asp or to emotion. Cleopatra observes her transition, though, and notes that it went "gently." So this seems to be a featureless fall. The Queen's own death cuts her speech off in mid-sentence, so there is no possibility that it will not be attended to. She speaks again of gentleness as the asp's poison takes effect, or as she presumes it must be taking effect:

> CLEOPATRA As sweet as balm, as soft as air, as gentle,—
> O Antony!—Nay, I will take thee too.
> [*Applying another asp to her arm.*]
> What should I stay—
> [*Dies*]
> CHARMIAN In this vild world? So, fare thee well!
> Now boast thee, death, in thy possession lies

A lass unparallel'd. Downy windows, close;
And golden Phoebus never be beheld
Of eyes again so royal! (5.2.311–18)

Charmian, attending her mistress loyally, completes her sentence and refers to one of the components of liveliness encountered above (but in reverse). It seems reasonable to assume that either the Queen's eyes have closed, or that her maid will now tenderly close them for her. Beyond this, not much is said except that again the death seems to be painless and the actor's challenge is to switch off the final signs in some palpable but dignified way. And the slump of the body into its throne, the lapse into unnatural stillness, the fixing of the face: these are all things that we simulate, I would argue, acting as well as experiencing. This is a moment where even to read the text is to imagine not just the way Cleopatra dies, but the way that a great actor would perform the moment.

The last death is Charmian's own. Here there is a greater sense of urgency, as the women have finally been interrupted by Roman guards. Nevertheless she has time to apply an asp:

1ST GUARD Caesar hath sent—
CHARMIAN Too slow a messenger.
[*Applies an asp.*]
O, come apace, dispatch! I partly feel thee.
1ST GUARD Approach ho, all's not well; Caesar's beguil'd.
2ND GUARD There's Dolabella sent from Caesar; call him.
1ST GUARD What work is here, Charmian? Is this well done?
CHARMIAN It is well done, and fitting for a princess
Descended of so many royal kings.
Ah, soldier! [*Charmian dies.*] (5.2.321–8)

Charmian is able to finish her sentences, and wishes for more speed. "I partly feel thee" suggests that she knows the poison is working but it has not yet taken her over. The final "Ah, soldier!" could be acted in many ways: is this pain, or grief, or a final breath, or something else, or a merger of several things? What is clear is that for the third time in the scene, a character has died in a particular, understated way on the stage, which allows the process of losing vitality to be encountered without being obscured by violence or frenzy.

In three more of Shakespeare's tragedies the performance of death takes on this quality because of a juxtaposition between the loss and the regaining of the basic aspects of life. In *Romeo and Juliet*, *King Lear* and *Othello*, plays separated by a decade or so in total, Shakespeare keeps coming back to the possibility or actuality of returning life, just at the play's most painful moments. Lear's last moments include an obsessive interest in the possibility that his dead daughter may actually be alive. He appeals to the familiar feather, and also to a mirror (where condensation would reveal breath), as means of testing:

KING LEAR I know when one is dead, and when one lives;
She's dead as earth. Lend me a looking-glass,
If that her breath will mist or stain the stone,
Why then she lives.
KENT Is this the promis'd end?
EDGAR Or image of that horror?
ALBANY Fall, and cease!
KING LEAR This feather stirs, she lives! If it be so,
It is a chance which does redeem all sorrows
That ever I have felt. (5.3.261–8)

Kent and Edgar are exclaiming at the awfulness of the scene in general—the precious daughter mourned by her abject father—but there may also be something special in the vain hope that makes it so utterly like the end. The deictic "This" suggests that this is a prop feather rather than an imaginary or insubstantial one, but on the other hand, there seems little need to imagine that Lear gets, or really needs, a mirror in response to his request, so perhaps the feather too is imaginary.[20]

"If it be so," of course, is a huge "if." Yet even as his own death becomes entirely imminent Lear is still reaching after the signs of life in his daughter. Again it is her mouth that occupies his attention.[21] The moment of his death is unclear, but one place editors put it is exactly at the point he is most insistent that Cordelia is breathing:

KING LEAR Do you see this? Look on her! Look her lips,
Look there, look there! [*He dies*]
EDGAR He faints. My lord, my lord!
KENT Break, heart, I prithee break!
EDGAR Look up, my lord.
KENT Vex not his ghost. O, let him pass, he hates him
That would upon the rack of this tough world
Stretch him out longer.
EDGAR He is gone, indeed. (5.3.311–16)

For the actor playing Lear, there is some space to perform the ebbing of life and the possibility that an optimistic thought is the King's last. I think the moment of dying covers everything from the "faint" (which has to be accompanied by a distinct action) and Edgar's realization that the King truly has no vital signs left, "gone indeed." Kent seems to pull Edgar away and the three lines of his speech seem deliberately to leave room for the audience to see the light finally going out.[22]

In the final scene of *Othello* there is a different (though also horrific) attentiveness to the evidence of life. Unlike in *King Lear*, there is some unexpected tenacity in a key character's vitality, but this does not help. As Othello closes in on the murder of his wife, he urges stillness:

> OTHELLO Peace, and be still!
> DESDEMONA I will so. What's the matter? (5.2.46–7)

As the scene unfolds this emphasis continues. Desdemona's actual and metaphorical mobility (her ability to leave him; her ability to transfer her affections; *la donna è mobile*) have proved intolerable, and now he brings an end to it. The moment of death is made chaotic by Emilia's interruption and Othello's uncertainty:

> OTHELLO What noise is this? Not dead? not yet quite dead?
> I that am cruel am yet merciful,
> I would not have thee linger in thy pain.
> So, so.
> EMILIA [*Within.*] What, ho! my lord, my lord!
> OTHELLO Who's there?
> EMILIA [*Within.*] O, good my lord, I would speak a word with you!
> OTHELLO Yes—'Tis Emilia.—By and by.—She's dead.
> 'Tis like she comes to speak of Cassio's death;
> The noise was here. Hah, no more moving?
> Still as the grave. Shall she come in? Were't good?
> I think she stirs again. No. What's best to do?
> If she come in, she'll sure speak to my wife.
> My wife, my wife! what wife? I have no wife. (5.2.86–97)

As with Hermione's statue, we don't know how to watch Desdemona. It is difficult to prove this, but my sense is that audiences don't simulate the experience of dying violently in the same way one might simulate the death of Cleopatra or the coming-to-life of Imogen. Nevertheless, we may still join Othello staring at Desdemona and looking for signs, but are we sympathetically disposed towards the actor such that we look for a convincing performance of death, or such that we look for some residual vitality? The hero's panic infects our attention, surely, so we are even less sure what to look for and what we are looking at. By the end, however, Othello has entirely convinced himself that Desdemona is dead and we have no reason to doubt it.

This makes it all the more strange and shocking that Desdemona revives briefly a few lines later. The actor has been subjected to close attention and has produced a satisfactory lack of vital signs. Now there has to be some sort of revival:

DESDEMONA	O, falsely, falsely murder'd!
EMILIA	O Lord, what cry is that?
OTHELLO	That? what?
EMILIA	Out, and alas, that was my lady's voice. Help, help, ho, help! O lady, speak again! Sweet Desdemona! O sweet mistress, speak!
DESDEMONA	A guiltless death I die.
EMILIA	O, who hath done this deed?
DESDEMONA	Nobody; I myself. Farewell Commend me to my kind lord. O, farewell! [*Dies*]
OTHELLO	Why, how should she be murd'red? (5.2.117–26)

It seems that Desdemona must be concealed from Emilia's view for a while here, and so the audience's attention may well simply not be on Desdemona as she revives. But the actor has to muster speech somehow, and that surely entails some sort of transformation back into theatrical life. Our ability to imagine what it must be like to be Desdemona here is compromised by the strange things she says: her inexplicably valiant (if that is what it is) decision to lie about her murder is hard to empathize with, and it seems as if she is in a strange cognitive state not unlike Imogen's. This time, Desdemona has final words and the space in which to expel her last breath ("O") while the other signs of life pass away. Second time around, unless the play is to descend into parody, it cannot be a false death.

The last example in this essay is the earliest of these tragic instances (preceded only among all the examples cited by the *Henry VI Part 3* feather). The revival of Juliet is perhaps paradigmatic for all the subsequent examples. Later revivals refuse the clarity and absoluteness of her tragic fate; later revisions seem to require some strange or ironic spin off its perfect poignancy. First Romeo encourages us to look closely at the dead body:

How oft when men are at the point of death
Have they been merry, which their keepers call
A lightning before death! O, how may I
Call this a lightning? O my love, my wife,
Death, that hath suck'd the honey of thy breath,
Hath had no power yet upon thy beauty:
Thou art not conquer'd; beauty's ensign yet
Is crimson in thy lips and in thy cheeks,
And death's pale flag is not advanced there. (5.3.88–96)

The potion is supposed to give an appearance of death, but it is not perfect. One of the signs of life, colour, is still there.[23] The actor lying there presumably has to minimize any signs of breath but does not have to *think pale* (or to wear any make-up to that effect). Romeo, however, is not led to doubt anything. It makes sense to him, perhaps, in his slightly giddy state, that Juliet's beauty cannot be extinguished. Romeo's death invites sensorimotor interactions in some complex ways:

O, here
Will I set up my everlasting rest,
And shake the yoke of inauspicious stars
From this world-wearied flesh. Eyes, look your last!
Arms, take your last embrace! and, lips, O you
The doors of breath, seal with a righteous kiss
A dateless bargain to engrossing death!
Come, bitter conduct, come, unsavoury guide!
Thou desperate pilot, now at once run on
The dashing rocks thy sea-sick weary bark!
Here's to my love! [*Drinks.*] O true apothecary!
Thy drugs are quick. Thus with a kiss I die. [*Dies.*] (5.3.109–20)

By addressing different parts of his body Romeo requires us, perhaps, to imagine (if not to simulate) how they might be switched off. A more vivid encounter comes when he takes the poison (with a toast, "here's to my love!"), and then feels the rapid effects. This is one of Shakespeare's most palpable encounters with the extinguishing of vital signs, because it invites us to think so specifically about a fatal process (more than Cleopatra's asp, which is always being glossed over, and its effects minimized). This is complicated and perhaps interrupted by the kiss: the audience knows that this is a heavily ironic meeting of life and death; but it is too late and also too early for Romeo to realize his error.

Then Juliet wakes up. The Friar comes in, sees dead bodies, noting with some irony that Romeo is already pale. Then he sees that (as he expects) Juliet is coming back to consciousness:

> FRIAR Romeo, O, pale! Who else? What, Paris too?
> And steep'd in blood? Ah, what an unkind hour
> Is guilty of this lamentable chance!
> The lady stirs.
> [*Juliet rises.*]
> JULIET O comfortable friar! where is my lord?
> I do remember well where I should be,
> And there I am. Where is my Romeo? (5.3.144–50)

"Stir" is again an important word: it denotes the basic mobility of a living thing. But Juliet's waking is not just a matter of moving: she has to recover all those other signs of life. In comparison with Imogen and Desdemona (who—to make the point again—are surely revisitations of the motif from this earlier play) she is remarkably self-possessed. In some ways it is psychologically more interesting to focus on disorientation, but this potion has its own unique effects, and Juliet's self-possession extends even so far as to lead her to wonder at her own self-possession.

There is a sharp detail when Juliet notices Romeo's body. She kisses him, and finds his lips are warm. Quickly she decides that her death must follow, and this is hastened by the arrival of the Watch:

> Yea, noise? Then I'll be brief. O happy dagger,
> [*Taking Romeo's dagger.*]
> This is thy sheath [*stabs herself*]; there rust, and let me die.
> [*Falls on Romeo's body, and dies.*] (5.3.169–70)

As a challenge for the actor this death is much simpler than her revivification shortly earlier, and it is also simpler than Romeo's death by poison. The violence of her suicide lets out her life in a more conventional way, and attention to vital signs is going to be less easy to sustain and direct and ponder. However, the cumulative effect of the scene, with its configurations and reconfigurations of movements into and out of deathliness, makes it another complex encounter with animation as a quality of life and theatre.

Shakespeare is not the only writer to depict the basic experiences of being alive in such a way as to make his audience—and readers too—think it through with every aspect of their intelligence. Timothy Harrison, for example, has described how Adam's sweat, the feeling of being in the sun, the way life feels before and after the Fall, and other signs, make up *Paradise Lost*'s interest in vitality.[24] However, the interpretative framework offered by the idea of kinesic intelligence offers a new perspective on Shakespeare's special attentiveness to the signs of animation arising from plots in which the boundary between life and death is explored in strange ways. While the approach illuminates the plays, recognizing the way in which they work on and with our minds, the plays in turn illuminate the approach. Kinesic intelligence needs to, because it can, reach beyond gestures, responses, and intentions, into the fainter fundamentals of life, things which are always with us but rarely perceived, signs that may be most accessible, and most strangely accessible, when we think through what it would take to perform them.

Notes

1. All Shakespeare quotations are from *The Riverside Shakespeare*, ed. G. Blakemore Evans, 2nd ed. (Boston: Houghton Mifflin, 1997).
2. Andrew Sofer, *The Stage Life of Props* (Ann Arbor: University of Michigan Press, 2003), and Marvin Carlson, *The Haunted Stage: The Theatre as Memory Machine* (Ann Arbor: University of Michigan Press, 2003) both describe the vivid lives of tangible props as they are passed from production to production. See also, more directly about the Shakespearean theatre, *Staged Properties in Early Modern England*, ed. Jonathan Gil Harris and Natasha Korda (Cambridge: Cambridge University Press, 2002). Some of this vividness applies even to the elusive feathers here.
3. Guillemette Bolens, *The Style of Gestures: Embodiment and Cognition in Literary Narrative* (Baltimore: Johns Hopkins University Press, 2012), 8, 9.
4. Terence Cave, *Thinking with Literature: Towards a Cognitive Criticism* (Oxford: Oxford University Press, 2016), 8.
5. As in Amy Cook, *Shakespearean Neuroplay: Reinvigorating the Study of Dramatic Texts and Performance Through Cognitive Science* (Basingstoke: Palgrave, 2010), and Bruce McConachie, *Engaging Audiences: A Cognitive Approach to Spectating in the Theatre* (Basingstoke: Palgrave, 2008).
6. See Hannah Chapelle Wojciehowski, "Statues That Move: Vitality Effects in *The Winter's Tale*," *Literature and Theology* 28 (2014): 299–315, and Ellen Spolsky's response, "Vitality Effects: Hidden in Plain View: A Response to Hannah Chapelle Wojciehowski," *Literature and Theology*

28 (2014): 316–320. I am also indebted to Penelope Woods, "The Audience of the Indoor Theatres," in *Moving Shakespeare Indoors: Performance and Repertoire in the Jacobean Playhouse*, ed. Andrew Gurr and Farah Karim-Cooper (Cambridge: Cambridge University Press, 2014), 152–67. Woods explores the ways in which different theatres (such as the Blackfriars, with its indoor intimacy) may have affected the ways in which audiences attended to onstage faces, movements, breaths, etc.

7. Wojciehowski has published some innovative research arising from her collaboration with one of the key figures in mirror neuron science, Vittorio Gallese. While in some ways the concept of "kinesic intelligence" as Bolens defines it aims to separate itself from this field (preferring to emphasise the application of a faculty rather than the consequences of an automatic response), these two pieces represent some rapprochement between this view of the humanities and the mirror neurons idea. See Hannah Wojciehowski and Vittorio Gallese, "How Stories Make Us Feel: Toward an Embodied Narratology," *California Italian Studies* 2 (2011), http://escholarship.org/uc/item/3jg726c2, and Hannah Chapelle Wojciehowski, "The Mirror Neuron Mechanism and Literary Studies: An Interview with Vittorio Gallese," *California Italian Studies* 2 (2010), http://escholarship.org/uc/item/56f8v9bv.
8. See Ellen Spolsky, *Word vs Image: Cognitive Hunger in Shakespeare's England* (Basingstoke: Palgrave, 2007).
9. Daniel Stern, *Forms of Vitality: Exploring Dynamic Experience in Psychology, the Arts, Psychotherapy, and Development* (Oxford: Oxford University Press, 2010).
10. Stern, 57–70; quoting p. 70.
11. Garrett A. Sullivan, Jr., *Sleep, Romance and Embodiment: Vitality from Spenser to Milton* (Cambridge: Cambridge University Press, 2012).
12. Antonio Damasio, *Descartes' Error: Emotion, Reason, and the Human Brain* (New York: Putnam, 1994).
13. See especially Evelyn Tribble "'Oh, She's Warm': Touch in *The Winter's Tale*," in *Knowing Shakespeare: Senses, Embodiment and Cognition*, ed. Lowell Gallagher and Shankar Raman (Basingstoke: Palgrave, 2010), 65–81. Tribble is especially good on the importance of the actor's body as part of the haptic scenario.
14. For an interesting take on the cognitive characteristics being shown here (and with reference to other later plays), see Jennifer Lewin, "'Your Actions Are My Dreams': Sleepy Minds in Shakespeare's Last Plays," *Shakespeare Studies* 31 (2003): 184–204, and also William Sherman, "Shakespearean Soliloquy: Sleepy Language and *The Tempest*," in *Renaissance Transformations: The Making of English Writing, 1500–1650*, ed. Tom Healy and Margaret Healy (Edinburgh: Edinburgh University Press, 2009), 177–91.

15. One of the interesting intertexts for the statue scene, the Alcestis story and Euripides' dramatic version thereof, brings the shadow of death into the picture. The statue may not be dead but one of its predecessors, Admetus's lost queen, was (until Heracles saved her). See Sarah Dewar-Watson, "The *Alcestis* and the Statue Scene in *The Winter's Tale*," *Shakespeare Quarterly* 60 (2009): 73–80.
16. See Kaara L. Peterson, "Shakespearean Revivification Narratives: Early Modern Undead," *Shakespeare Studies* 32 (2004): 40–66, and also Peterson's *Popular Medicine, Hysterical Disease, and Social Controversy in Shakespeare's England* (Farnham: Ashgate, 2010).
17. Edward Jorden, *A Briefe Discourse of a Disease Called the Suffocation of the Mother* (London: John Windet, 1603), D2r.
18. Michael de Montaigne, *The Essayes or Morall, Politike and Millitarie Discourses*, trans. John Florio (London: Edward Blount, 1603), E3r.
19. Pedro de Soto, *The Maner to Dye Well: An Introduction Most Compendiouslie Shewinge the Fruytfull Remembrance of the Last Fowre Things: That is to Say, Death, Hel, Judgement, and the Joyes of Heaven* (London: Richard Jones, 1578), D5r–D5v.
20. See Amy Cook, "If: Lear's Feather and the Staging of Science," in *The Return of Theory in Early Modern English Studies: Tarrying with the Subjunctive*, ed. Paul Cefalu and Bryan Reynolds (New York: Palgrave Macmillan, 2011), 48–68.
21. This moment, and especially the way that speech and character are related, are illuminated by Michael Holahan, "'Look, Her Lips': Softness of Voice, Construction of Character in *King Lear*," *Shakespeare Quarterly* 4 (1997): 406–31.
22. For the idea that this death occurs too late, that Lear has "over-lived," see Emily Wilson, *Mocked with Death: Tragic Overliving from Sophocles to Milton* (Baltimore: Johns Hopkins University Press, 2004).
23. See Tanya Pollard, "'A Thing Like Death': Sleeping Potions and Poisons in *Romeo and Juliet* and *Antony and Cleopatra*," *Renaissance Drama* 32 (2003): 95–121.
24. Timothy Harrison, "Adamic Awakening and the Feeling of Being Alive in Paradise Lost," *Milton Studies* 54 (2013): 29–58.

Bibliography

Blakemore Evans, Gwynne, ed. *The Riverside Shakespeare*, 2nd ed. Boston: Houghton Mifflin, 1997.

Bolens, Guillemette. *The Style of Gestures: Embodiment and Cognition in Literary Narrative*. Baltimore: Johns Hopkins University Press, 2012.

Carlson, Marvin. *The Haunted Stage: The Theatre as Memory Machine*. Ann Arbor: University of Michigan Press, 2003.

Cave, Terence. *Thinking with Literature: Towards a Cognitive Criticism*. Oxford: Oxford University Press, 2016.

Cook, Amy. *Shakespearean Neuroplay: Reinvigorating the Study of Dramatic Texts and Performance Through Cognitive Science*. Basingstoke: Palgrave, 2010.

———. If: Lear's Feather and the Staging of Science. In *The Return of Theory in Early Modern English Studies: Tarrying with the Subjunctive*, edited by Paul Cefalu and Bryan Reynolds. New York: Palgrave Macmillan, 2011.

Damasio, Antonio. *Descartes' Error: Emotion, Reason, and the Human Brain*. New York: Putnam, 1994.

Dewar-Watson, Sarah. The *Alcestis* and the Statue Scene in *The Winter's Tale*. *Shakespeare Quarterly* 60 (2009): 73–80.

Gil Harris, Jonathan and Natasha Korda, eds. *Staged Properties in Early Modern England*. Cambridge: Cambridge University Press, 2002.

Harrison, Timothy. Adamic Awakening and the Feeling of Being Alive in Paradise Lost. *Milton Studies* 54 (2013): 29–58.

Holahan, Michael. 'Look, Her Lips': Softness of Voice, Construction of Character in *King Lear*. *Shakespeare Quarterly* 4 (1997): 406–31.

Jorden, Edward. *A Briefe Discourse of a Disease Called the Suffocation of the Mother*. London: John Windet, 1603.

Lewin, Jennifer. 'Your Actions Are My Dreams': Sleepy Minds in Shakespeare's Last Plays. *Shakespeare Studies* 31 (2003): 184–204.

McConachie, Bruce. *Engaging Audiences: A Cognitive Approach to Spectating in the Theatre*. Basingstoke: Palgrave, 2008.

Montaigne, Michael de. *The Essayes or Morall, Politike and Millitarie Discourses*. Translated by John Florio. London: Edward Blount, 1603.

Peterson, Kaara L. Shakespearean Revivification Narratives: Early Modern Undead. *Shakespeare Studies* 32 (2004): 40–66.

———. *Popular Medicine, Hysterical Disease, and Social Controversy in Shakespeare's England*. Farnham: Ashgate, 2010.

Pollard, Tanya. 'A Thing like Death': Sleeping Potions and Poisons in *Romeo and Juliet* and *Antony and Cleopatra*. *Renaissance Drama* 32 (2003): 95–121.

Sherman, William. Shakespearean Soliloquy: Sleepy Language and *The Tempest*. In *Renaissance Transformations: The Making of English Writing, 1500–1650*, edited by Tom Healy and Margaret Healy, 177–91. Edinburgh: Edinburgh University Press, 2009.

Sofer, Andrew. *The Stage Life of Props*. Ann Arbor: University of Michigan Press, 2003.

Soto, Pedro de. *The Maner to Dye Well: An Introduction Most Compendiouslie Shewinge the Fruytfull Remembrance of the Last Fowre Things: That Is to Say, Death, Hel, Judgement, and the Joyes of Heaven*. London: Richard Jones, 1578.

Spolsky, Ellen. *Word vs Image: Cognitive Hunger in Shakespeare's England*. Basingstoke: Palgrave, 2007.

———. Vitality Effects: Hidden in Plain View: A Response to Hannah Chapelle Wojciehowski. *Literature and Theology* 28 (2014): 316–320.

Stern, Daniel. *Forms of Vitality: Exploring Dynamic Experience in Psychology, the Arts, Psychotherapy, and Development*. Oxford: Oxford University Press, 2010.

Sullivan, Garrett A., Jr. *Sleep, Romance and Embodiment: Vitality from Spenser to Milton*. Cambridge: Cambridge University Press, 2012.

Tribble, Evelyn. 'Oh, She's Warm': Touch in *The Winter's Tale*. In *Knowing Shakespeare: Senses, Embodiment and Cognition*, edited by Lowell Gallagher and Shankar Raman, 65–81. Basingstoke: Palgrave, 2010.

Wilson, Emily. *Mocked with Death: Tragic Overliving from Sophocles to Milton*. Baltimore: Johns Hopkins University Press, 2004.

Wojciehowski, Hannah Chapelle. The Mirror Neuron Mechanism and Literary Studies: An Interview with Vittorio Gallese. *California Italian Studies* 2 (2010). http://escholarship.org/uc/item/56f8v9bv

———. Statues that Move: Vitality Effects in *The Winter's Tale*. *Literature and Theology* 28 (2014): 299–315.

Wojciehowski, Hannah, and Vittorio Gallese. How Stories Make Us Feel: Toward an Embodied Narratology. *California Italian Studies* 2 (2011). http://escholarship.org/uc/item/3jg726c2

Woods, Penelope. The Audience of the Indoor Theatres. In *Moving Shakespeare Indoors: Performance and Repertoire in the Jacobean Playhouse*, edited by Andrew Gurr and Farah Karim-Cooper, 152–67. Cambridge: Cambridge University Press, 2014.

CHAPTER 11

Kinesic Intelligence on the Early Modern English Stage

Evelyn Tribble

In her ground-breaking work *The Style of Gestures: Embodiment and Cognition in Literary Narrative*, Guillemette Bolens takes up the topic of kinesic intelligence, adopting Ellen Spolsky's definition of the concept as "the human capacity to discern and interpret body movement, body postures, gestures, and facial expressions in real situations, as well as in our reception of visual art."[1] In Bolens's discussion of literary narrative, this capacity is mediated from writer to reader through written language: "Kinesic intelligence in literature is the faculty that enables us to produce and use perceptual simulations in order to understand narrated movements and gestures."[2] Bolens argues that readers' embodied kinesic intelligence, grounded in the body, allows them to grasp the complex kinesics of the literary text, to raise it from the two-dimensional into the fully realized world of the imagination. Bolens charts a kind of resonance between readers' bodies and the writer's words, expressed through the skilled representation of gesture. Readers of Jane Austen's *Sense and Sensibility*, for example, recognize the contrast between Marianne's unguarded twitches and facial expression that betray her feelings to Elinor's carefully regulated

E. Tribble (✉)
University of Otago, Dunedin, New Zealand

K. Banks, T. Chesters (eds.), *Movement in Renaissance Literature*, Cognitive Studies in Literature and Performance,
https://doi.org/10.1007/978-3-319-69200-5_11

face and body as she struggles to govern herself. Austen makes plain the "physiological cost of Elinor's self-command."[3] Bolens provides a way of reading such moments that goes beyond simply analysing the "cultural and epistemological conventions associated with non-verbal communication"[4]; in particular, her work on the sensorimotor and cognitive elements of literature moves towards a fully embodied theory of reading.

As Bolens shows, researchers in gesture have demonstrated that spoken language is inherently multi-modal, employing both gesture and speech. Gesture is not mere hand-waving, but plays an active causal role in thought and in language production. The work of Susan Goldin-Meadow and David McNeill, amongst many others, has clearly demonstrated the tight links between the brain and the hand.[5] In comparison to the rich multi-modal nature of the hand-speech-nervous system link in face-to face interactions, the skilled narrative artists whom Bolens discusses have only written language at their disposal. Thus, they face the challenge of reanimating the attenuated forms of language available in written form, that is, they must repurpose it and reinvigorate the written word with the immediacy and multi-modality of gesture. The craft and skill needed to create a believable—and animate—world on paper is amply borne out by the fictional examples Bolens scrutinizes.

When we move from the realm of the novel into the realm of theatre, we introduce another agent into this nexus of skill: the trained actor. I argue that foregrounding the relationship between skill and kinesis can help to refine and broaden the model of kinesic intelligence put forward by Bolens and Spolsky. Bolens usefully employs Shaun Gallagher's description of bodily schema, which he defines as a largely pre-noetic "system of sensory-motor processes that constantly regulate posture and movement [...] without reflective awareness or the necessity of perceptual monitoring."[6] Gallagher here distinguishes conscious, reflective movement—such as one might undertake when learning how to dribble a basketball or how to swing a racquet—from the relatively unreflective actions we perform when, for instance, we adjust our body when picking up an object. This is a crucial distinction, but there is much more to skilled movement than the pre-noetic/noetic divide. Bolens recognizes this point in her discussion of the trained body of the dancer. Shaping the body over time through training and experience is above all the job of experts in movement such as actors and dancers, who of necessity must bring the everyday movements of their bodies into conscious awareness, just as skilled writers learn to capture movements in words. A full study of kinesic intelligence requires examining how "the acquisition of skill shapes the body," in the words of neuroanthropologist Greg Downey.[7]

In early modern theatre, the trained body of the actor mediates the kinesic skill of the playwright. The player, above all, is an expert in movement and animation. I have written elsewhere about the particular form of trained movement known as action in the early modern period—to call this form of bodily intelligence only gesture understates how crucial it was in the early modern period. It is not, as is sometimes thought, a mere decoration or a holdover from outmoded forms of acting, but is instead a key manifestation of the mindful body. The playwright's words are taken into body, animated through the spirits of the actor, and communicated—in a literal sense—to the audience. In the *Passions of the Mind in Generall*, Thomas Wright described action as "visible eloquence," which aptly captures the yoking of the mind and body that was the pinnacle of the actor's art.[8]

In his *Apology for Actors*, Thomas Heywood argues that the skilled action gives the actor a direct hold over the audience, allowing him to "mooue the spirits of the beholder to admiration."[9] As Joseph Roach has pointed out, the animation of the actor kindles a reciprocating action in the spectator, a resonance of spirits that cannot be attained through word or image alone.[10] For Heywood, action is the *sine qua non* of the actor; rhetorical treatises prescribe that the orator must be skilled in the traditional disciplines of invention, disposition, elocution, memory and pronunciation, "yet all are imperfect without the sixth, which is Action; for be his invention neuer so fluent and exquisite, his disposition and order neuer so composed and formall, his eloquence, and elaborate phrases, neuer so materiall and pithy, his memory neuer so firme and retentitue, his pronuntiation neuer so musicall and plausive, yet without a comely and elegant gesture, a gratious and bewitching kind of action. I hold all the rest as nothing."[11]

These are of course interested accounts, arguments made by defenders of the stage against its detractors. But they nevertheless capture something of the framework of values that governed the stage, and the sense of distinctively kinesic intelligence brought to bear by the actor upon his part, as well as the way that such kinesis reverberates through the theatre to affect the spectator, a sharing of the animating spirits between actor and viewer. The ability to command "grace" was seen as the chief distinguishing feature of the truly skilled player. In *Richard II*, the Duke of York describes the entry of Bolingbroke and the deposed Richard into London; Bolingbroke, on his horse, commands the "greedy looks" (5.2.13) of the crowds, whilst "men's eyes/did scowl on Richard":

As in a theatre the eyes of men,
After a well-grac'd actor leaves the stage,
Are idly bent on him that enters next,
Thinking his prattle to be tedious. (5.2.23–26)

The training needed to produce such effects began early. The early modern theatre employed an apprentice system, in which boys were bound to adult players in formal or informal fashion. These boys practised increasingly complex forms of kinesic intelligence, beginning with the simple act of walking on stage, which is considerably more difficult than it seems. Boys who came to the stage with some form of grammar school training were no doubt adept at remembering verses, but the development of situation awareness—the composure needed to simply to stand on stage—was developed over years. Shakespeare humorously comments on the training that underpinned the development of kinesic intelligence in *Love's Labour's Lost*, in which young Moth is painstakingly coached to deliver a speech to the ladies: "Action and accent they did teach him there:/'Thus must thou speak and thus thy body bear'" (5.2.99–100). This description parodies the painstaking training of boys in the adult companies, who were taught to grace their parts by integrating voice and movement. Through their training in kinesic intelligence, young actors learned to lift the pre-noetic into conscious awareness, to transform untrained gesticulations into graceful intentional movements to attract the eyes and attention of the audience.

Boys were also trained in very distinct forms of kinesic intelligence: they specialized in playing women and, in the children's companies, old men. What has been called the transvestite stage has garnered enormous critical attention, of course, and Shakespeare and other playwrights often call attention to the different forms of kinesis needed to portray the cross-dressed boy. In *The Merchant of Venice*, Portia tells Nerissa that when they "turn to men":

I'll wear my dagger with the braver grace
And speak between the change of man and boy
With a reed voice, and turn two mincing steps
Into a manly stride. (3.4.62–5)

This comment playfully invokes and enacts the kinesic skills displayed by boys playing women's parts on the early modern stage. The boy playing Portia has up to this point performed a woman's part relatively invisibly;

here, however, as the character announces the intention to don male disguise, the young player demonstrates his ability to code-switch between feminine and masculine bodily dispositions. Similarly, in the Induction to *Antonio and Mellida*, the boys are "perfect"—they know the words of their parts by heart—but they are unsure of how to approach the animation of their characters. To play a Duke Piero is advised:

> O, ho: then thus frame your exterior shape,
> To haughty form of elate majesty;
> As if you held the palsy shaking-head
> Of reeling chance under your fortune's belt,
> In strictest vassalage grow big in thought,
> As swollen with glory of successful arms. (Ind. 5–10)

This part is relatively simple—"Who can not be proud, stroke up the hair, and strut!"—but Antonio is flummoxed at having to play both a male and female part in the same play: "Aye but when use hath taught me action, to hit the right point of a lady's part, I shall grow ignorant when I must turne young Prince againe, how but to truss my hose." (Ind 81–3).

These meta-theatrical references provide a sense of the appeal of boy actors: the disparity between their physical bodies and the varieties and skills of kinesis that animated them. A parallel from contemporary viewing habits might illuminate this point. In 2005 the late Philip Seymour Hoffman's impersonation of Truman Capote came in for enormous praise, not despite but *because* of the huge disparity in size between Capote and Hoffman. A critical response was:

> Talk about alchemy! When I heard he was cast, I was skeptical, because he's so much bigger than Capote. Hoffman reportedly listened to many tapes of Capote and sometimes when gifted and porous actors faithfully duplicate the stammers and pauses and delicate rhythms of their subjects, they get inside those subjects' heads—they become possessed. That's what obviously happened here: Hoffman goes beyond the surface mannerisms and diction. He disappears into Capote.[12]

This act disappearance earned Hoffman the Best Actor Academy Award in 2006, a confirmation of the well-known maxim that biopics are certain paths to an Oscar. This genre allows critics and audiences to evaluate how the actor negotiates the gap between the historical body and mannerisms of the subject and his or her own body, as mediated by his or her own celebrity. When the gaps are, or are perceived to be especially wide—the imposing Hoffman playing the diminutive Capote—the actors' skill is seen as correspondingly impressive. It is perhaps for this reason that one of the most prized skills of boy players on the early modern stage was the ability to embody old men.

While boys playing women have received enormous attention, much less scholarship has focused on boys performing what Lucy Munro has called "age transvestitism."[13] Children's companies throughout the period featured boys playing old men. The most famous reference to this practice is Ben Jonson's "Epigram 120."[14] In this poem, Jonson mourns the death of Salomon Pavy, the child actor who "so did thrive / In grace and feature" that "Heaven and Nature seemed to strive / Which owned the creature." Jonson's conceit in the poem is that Pavy was so skilled at playing old men that the Fates mistook his age and took him before his time:

> [He] did act (what now we moan)
> Old men so duly,
> As, sooth, the Parcae thought him one,
> He played so truly.
> So, by error, to his fate
> They all consented.

As Munro notes, "When the children's companies were revived in 1599–1600, one of the aspects which seems to have most impressed their contemporaries was their performance of age."[15] If the disparity between the female character and the "boy beneath" attracted attention, so too did the disparity between the boy or youthful actor and the old man.

Boys who play old men invoke the familiar stereotype of the *senex*.[16] This trope is invoked when Hamlet rudely tells Polonius that "the satirical rogue says here that old men have grey beards, that their faces are wrinkled, their eyes purging thick amber and plum-tree gum, and that they have a plentiful lack of wit, together with most weak hams" (12.2. 96–200). With the plentiful lack of wit is a concomitant prolixity of speech. Perhaps the most famous description of age is Jacques' account of the "lean and slipper'd pantaloons" in the seven ages of man speech:

> With spectacles on nose, and pouch on side,
> His youthful hose well sav'd, a world too wide
> For his shrunk shank, and his big manly voice,
> Turning again toward childish treble, pipes
> And whistles in his sound. (*As You Like It* 2.7. 158–63)

In her discussion of the voice and masculinity on the early modern stage, Gina Bloom argues that Jacques's speech links the boy, yet to generate enough heat for full maturity, to the old man, shrunken into a parody of a child.[17] This is both a progressive and recursive journey—the old man "sans teeth" like the mewling infant, the pantaloon with his sparse hair, shrill voice and thin hams like the boy. So boys bear physiological homologies not just to women, but to elderly men.

As Munro has argued, and as the Jonson poem confirms, the plays performed by companies such as the Children of Queen's Revels reveal a particular fascination with such playing across age—or age transvestitism. It seems to have been thought of not just as a shtick good for a few laughs, but as an art of interest in its own right, just as the art of portraying women might command attention. The work of John Marston is a particularly complex portrayal of the working across age lines; his 1604 play *The Fawn* reveals a sophisticated and witty examination of youth and age, as well as an interest in pushing the boundaries of skill of the boys and youths playing old men.

The plot of *The Fawn* revolves around Hercules, the Duke of Ferrara, later disguised as the Fawn (or parasitical courtier). Hercules has travelled to the Court of Urbino, where he disguises himself to watch his son, Tiberio, woo in his name the lovely Dulcimel, the daughter of the Duke of Urbino, Gonzago. So the play pits two elderly characters, Hercules and Gonzaga, against the youth Tiberio and the 15-year-old Dulcimel. All these characters are, of course, played by "children": the boys of the Children of the Queen's Revels. The ages of the young actors probably ranged from the early to the late teens.

Marston presents two distinct types of the elderly man. In writing Gonzago's part, he self-consciously parodies Polonius in *Hamlet*. Gonzago is full of saws, adages and advice, is easily distracted by rhetorical reflections, and is unwittingly made the dupe of Dulcimel's plotting to marry Tiberio rather than Hercules. As Charles Cathcart notes, Marston writes the part in direct imitation of Polonius, although Gonzago remains a comic butt rather than a victim.[18] Dulcimel is a much cannier and wilier version of Ophelia crossed with a comic Desdemona, well aware that it is up to her to initiate and orchestrate the love match with the hapless yet handsome Tiberio. These parallels and parodies are made especially evident in Gonzaga's advice to Dulcimel:

> Daughter, for that our last speech leaves the firmest print, be thus advised. When young Tiberio negotiates his father's love, hold heedy guard over thy passions, and still keep this full thought firm in thy reason: 'tis his old father's love the young man moves—[to GRANUFFO]—is't not well thought my lord; we must bear brain—and when thou shalt behold Tiberios life-full eyes and well-filled veins, complexion firm, and hair that curls with strength of lusty moisture—[to GRANUFFO] I think we yet can speak, we ha' been eloquent—thou must shape thy thoughts
> To apprehend his father well in years,
> A grave wise prince, whose beauty is his honour
> And well-passed life, and do not give thy thoughts
> Least liberty to shape a divers scope—
> My Lord Granuffo, pray ye note my phrase—
> So shalt thou not abuse thy younger hope,
> Nor afflict us…. (1.2.83–100)

Marston writes the part in the familiar prolix and rambling style of the *senex*, full of clauses, advice, digressions and asides. The overblown and digressive language signals the kinesic style to be adopted by the boy playing Gonzago. The character speaks in proverbs and the old-fashioned style of antitheses and balance. The adages are punctuated by self-congratulatory asides directed at the even more elderly "silent lord" Granuffo. The language, then, cues a particular kinesic style: the character fills out the clauses somatically.

Despite or perhaps because of its familiarity, the role demands complex and multiple levels of skill; and the distinctive kinesic intelligence displayed perhaps reflects some of the pleasures of disparity evident in the response to Philip Seymour Hoffman. The boy playing Gonzago is not simply presenting the familiar foibles of old age, but also produces an uncanny Polonius impression. This adds a delicious layer to the boy's performance, which almost certainly would mimic for knowledgeable spectators the physical signature of the King's Men player who portrayed him. The audience thus sees the distinctive style of the parodied actor displayed, despite the very different physique of the younger actor. Memories of movements or physical signatures can be remarkably enduring; I can vividly recall the peculiar batting stances and bodily twitches of dozens of baseball players of the 1980s, and as Will West reminds us, these physical quirks could constitute a kind of somatic intertextuality that seems to have been widespread on the early modern stage.[19]

Hercules represents a rather different approach to the old man. He walks on stage as a Duke, quite likely using the kinesic style alluded to in *Antonio and Mellida:* "Who can not be proud, stroke up the hair, and strut!" He divests himself of his ducal robes:

> And now, thou ceremonious sovereignty
> Ye proud, severer, stateful complements,
> The secret arts of rule—I put you off;
> Nor ever shall those manacles of form
> Once more lock up the appetite of blood. (1.1.36–40)

As he casts off his robes, the boy playing the part must also embody "repressed heat" and "wild longings" that Hercules has been forced to hide under the cover of a "steady life" as Duke (1.2.46, 55). Having laid aside "the manacles of form"—the ceremonial costume and state owing to his status as Duke—he enters Urbino disguised and is privy to his son Tiberio's attempt to woo Dulcimel on his behalf. The wooing-by-proxy scene centres around a pitiless scrutiny of a portrait of Hercules, apparently painted some years earlier, produced to convince Dulcimel of Hercules' vitality:

> DULCIMEL. Is this your father's true proportion? *Shows a picture*
> TIBERIO. No, lady, but the perfect counterfeit.
> DULCIMEL. And the best grac'd—
> TIBERIO. The painter's art could yield.
> DULCIMEL. I wonder he would send a counterfeit
> To move our love [...]
> TIBERIO. Why, fairest princess, if your eye dislike
> That deader piece, behold me his true form
> And livelier image; such my father hath been. [...]
> DULCIMEL. But is your Father's age thus fresh, hath yet his head
> So many hairs?
> TIBERIO. More, more, by many a one.
> DULCIMEL. More say you?
> TIBERIO. More.
> DULCIMEL. Right, sir, for this hath none.
> Is his eye so quick as this same piece makes him show?
> TIBERIO. The courtesy of art hath given more life to that part
> than the sad cares of state would grant my father.
> DULCIMEL. This model speaks about forty.

TIBERIO. Then doth it somewhat flatter, for our father hath seen more years, and is a little shrunk from the full strength of time.
GONZAGO. Somewhat coldly praised. (1.2.107–11; 130–40)

Having witnessed this event, Hercules then (disguised) hears the courtiers rehash it, in predictably exaggerated fashion:

By this light, I'll swear he [Tiberio] said his father had the hipgout, the strangury, the fistula *in ano*, and a most unabideable breath, no teeth, less eyes, great fingers, little legs, an eternal flux, and an everlasting cough of the lungs … threescore and five, to have and to hold, a lady of fifteen! (1.2.193–6, 200)

Afterwards, alone on stage, Hercules announces: "I never knew till now, how old I was" (1.2.318). Realizing that he himself has been the dupe of courtly flatterers, he vows revenge against such deceivers and to.

…waste this most prodigious heat,
That falls into my age, like scorching flames
In depth of numbed December, in flattering all
In all of their extremest viciousness. (1.2.345–8)

"I never knew till now how old I was," is a poignant and complicated sentiment. The roles of Gonzaga and especially Hercules demand enormous kinesic intelligence on the part of the young actors. For the boy/youth playing Hercules, the role is sedimented in a different and perhaps even more challenging fashion than that of Gonzago, especially as it works through multiple layers of disguise. In Munro's phrase, Hercules is a "superannuated prodigal" whose role exploits the liminal status of the boy actor. As discussed above, in the age system of the early modern period, the boy/youth bears some natural affinities to the old man he portrays. Yet the young actor portraying Hercules, like the boy playing Tiberio, would no doubt have "life-full eyes and well filled veins, complexion firm, and hair that curls with strength of lusty moisture." He must credibly portray an old man still full of vigour—as well as the painful, poignant and comic realization that such vigour is simply a delusion. The kinesic intelligence needed to work across such distinctive physical signatures is a hallmark of the achievements of the early modern stage.

Notes

1. Spolsky, "Elaborated Knowledge: Reading Kinesis in Pictures," *Poetics Today* 17 (1996): 157–80.
2. Bolens, *The Style of Gestures: Embodiment and Cognition in Literary Narrative* (Baltimore, MD: Johns Hopkins University Press, 2012), 19.
3. John Wiltshire, *Jane Austen and the Body: "The Picture of Health"* (Cambridge England; New York: Cambridge University Press, 1992), 36.
4. Bolens, *Style of Gestures*, 10.
5. Susan Goldin-Meadow, *Hearing Gesture: How our Hands Help Us Think* (Cambridge, Harvard University Press, 2005) and David McNeill, *Hand and Mind: What Gestures Reveal About Thought* (Chicago: University of Chicago Press, 1992).
6. Gallagher, *How the Body Shapes the Mind* (Oxford: Clarendon Press, 2005), 37.
7. Downey, "Educating the Eyes: Biocultural Anthropology and Physical Education," *Anthropology in Action* 12 (2005): 58.
8. Wright, *The Passions of the Mind in General* (London: 1604), M8v.
9. Heywood, "An Apology for Actors (1612)," in *Shakespeare's Theater: A Sourcebook*, ed. Tanya Pollard (Oxford: Blackwell Publishing, 2004), 213–54.
10. Roach, *The Player's Passion: Studies in the Science of Acting* (Ann Arbor: University of Michigan Press, 1985).
11. Heywood, "Apology for Actors."
12. David Edelstein, "The Truman Show Philip Seymour Hoffman's Brilliant Capote," http://www.slate.com/articles/arts/movies/2005/09/the_truman_show.html.
13. Munro, *Children of the Queen's Revels* (Cambridge: Cambridge University Press, 2005).
14. Jonson, "Epigram 120," in *The Cambridge Edition of the Works of Ben Jonson*, ed. David Bevington, Martin Butler and Ian Donaldson (Cambridge: Cambridge University Press, 2012), 5: 182–3.
15. Munro, *Children of the Queen's Revels.*
16. Doris V. Falk, "Proverbs and the Polonius Destiny," *Shakespeare Quarterly* 18 (1967): 28.
17. Gina Bloom, *Voice in Motion: Staging Gender, Shaping Sound in Early Modern England* (Philadelphia: University of Pennsylvania Press, 2007), 44.
18. Cathcart, "Borrowings and the Authorial Domain: Gostanzo, Polonius, and Marston's Gonzago," *Comparative Drama* 37 (2003): 159–174.
19. William N. West, "Intertheatricality," in *Early Modern Theatricality*, ed. Henry S. Turner (Oxford: Oxford University Press, 2013), 151–72.

Bibliography

Bloom, Gina. *Voice in Motion: Staging Gender, Shaping Sound in Early Modern England*. Philadelphia: University of Pennsylvania Press, 2007.

Bolens, Guillemette. *The Style of Gestures: Embodiment and Cognition in Literary Narrative*. Baltimore, MD: Johns Hopkins University Press, 2012.

Cathcart, Charles. Borrowings and the Authorial Domain: Gostanzo, Polonius, and Marston's Gonzago. *Comparative Drama* 37, no. 2 (2003): 159–74.

Downey, Greg. Educating the Eyes: Biocultural Anthropology and Physical Education. *Anthropology in Action* 12, no. 2 (2005): 56–71.

Edelstein, David. The Truman Show Philip Seymour Hoffman's Brilliant Capote, 2005. http://www.slate.com/articles/arts/movies/2005/09/the_truman_show.html

Falk, Doris V. Proverbs and the Polonius Destiny. *Shakespeare Quarterly* 18, no. 1 (1967): 23–36.

Gallagher, Shaun. *How the Body Shapes the Mind*. Oxford: Clarendon Press, 2005.

Goldin-Meadow, Susan. *Hearing Gesture: How Our Hands Help Us Think*. Cambridge: Harvard University Press, 2005.

Heywood, Thomas. An Apology for Actors (1612). In *Shakespeare's Theater: A Sourcebook*, edited by Tanya Pollard, 213–54. Oxford: Blackwell Publishing, 2004.

Jonson, Ben. Epigram 120. In *The Cambridge Edition of the Works of Ben Jonson*, edited by David Bevington, Martin Butler and Ian Donaldson, vol. 5. 182–3. Cambridge: Cambridge University Press, 2012.

Marston, John. *The Parasitaster, or The Fawn*. Edited by David A. Blostein. Manchester: Manchester University Press, 1978.

———. *Antonio and Mellida*. Edited by W. Reavely Gair. Manchester: Manchester University Press, 2004.

McNeill, David. *Hand and Mind: What Gestures Reveal About Thought*. Chicago: University of Chicago Press, 1992.

Munro, Lucy. *Children of the Queen's Revels*. Cambridge: Cambridge University Press, 2005.

Roach, Joseph R. *The Player's Passion: Studies in the Science of Acting*. Ann Arbor: University of Michigan Press, 1985.

Shakespeare, William. *The Arden Shakespeare Complete Works*. Edited by Richard Proudfoot, Ann Thompson and David Scott Kastan. London: Arden Shakespeare, 2011.

Spolsky, Ellen. Elaborated Knowledge: Reading Kinesis in Pictures. *Poetics Today* 17 (1996): 157–80.

West, William N. Intertheatricality. In *Early Modern Theatricality*, edited by Henry S. Turner, 151–72. Oxford: Oxford University Press, 2013.

Wiltshire, John. *Jane Austen and the Body: "The Picture of Health."* Cambridge England; New York: Cambridge University Press, 1992.

Wright, Thomas. *The Passions of the Mind in General*. London, 1604.

CHAPTER 12

How Do Audiences Act?

Ellen Spolsky

The Janus face of many of the essays in this collection puzzled me at first. While studying kinesis in Renaissance texts—an undertaking so new that there isn't yet an accepted vocabulary to describe the work—many of the authors here designate their discoveries in terms of classical rhetoric. Metaphor is the term that appears most frequently, but apostrophe, catachresis, anagnorisis, hypotyposis, chiasmus and anthimeria are also used to link new configurations to familiar categories. I had thought, rather, that instead of looking backward, the job these readers had undertaken was to investigate what the current cognitive sciences can tell us about how bodies make best use of the texts we value because they do *not* fit easily into what is already known.

But now I think I see the point. Classical rhetoric, back before it was reduced to a list of writerly possibilities or tropes, was indeed about producing motor resonance. As Chaim Perelman described it, rhetoric was always about people getting others to agree with them, or to do what they wanted done. The skilled orator used language instead of physical force.[1] The study of rhetoric, then, became a way of accounting for the overlap between the practice of skilled speakers and the simulated or mimetic use of oratory in imaginative texts and in the dramatic and plastic arts. The

E. Spolsky (✉)
Bar-Ilan University, Ramat Gan, Israel

K. Banks, T. Chesters (eds.), *Movement in Renaissance Literature*, Cognitive Studies in Literature and Performance, https://doi.org/10.1007/978-3-319-69200-5_12

terms traditionally used to describe the varieties of verbal persuasion, thus, have always been indirectly linked to the lived reality of readers' or audiences' bodies, and the study of those terms can be seen to have aimed, since its origins, at a description of how different forms of speech were assumed to influence the bodily states of their audiences. They would, thus, be signs (though, alas, hardly transparent ones), of the desires and intentions, beliefs and emotions of both speaker and hearer.[2]

In the spirit, then, of the authors here who have looked backward to move forward, I intend this afterword to advance further work on kinesis by reconnecting to some of what has already been written about how the forms of fiction appeal to what human bodies know about action, how words pull readers into their imagined worlds by engaging audiences' kinesic intelligence. This work has been interestingly enriched by recent neuroscientific approaches to brain processing that point a direction for the further development of this project. I am spurred on to this bidirectional undertaking by the most recent book on my desk about thinking and acting, Andy Clark's *Surfing Uncertainty: Prediction, Action, and the Embodied Mind*, in which a predictive processing model is expounded.[3] Clark surveys empirical work supporting a hypothesis describing brain work as an arrangement of hierarchical feedforward and feedback loops. The bidirectionality of our brains, on this view, produces "pansurprisingness" (91) as it guides our guesses about how our bodies will need to act in the face of what is about to happen. For that coinage alone he deserves our attention.

The predictive model unseats assumptions, made at least since John Locke, that consider the brain to be a rational operator, collecting information and acting when sufficient data has accumulated. It is instead proposed that the brain works by back and forth exchanges that produce possibilities from memories of experience that suggest what kinds of information should be searched for among the external arrays. The brain does not collect and analyse; it acts on guesses and corrects for errors, with a systematic and unavoidable uncertainty that must be accounted for in the processes that align already-in-place with new experience. I will mention as well the work of Leonhard Schilbach and colleagues, whose programmatic article of 2013, "Toward a second-person neuroscience," argues the need to move away from the model currently predominating in neuropsychology in which descriptions are produced by a detached and passive observer, a third-person cognizer, as it were.[4] In this model—and consistent with the predictive processing hypothesis—knowledge is understood as situated in the embodied interactions among people, producing a "study of real-time social encounters in a truly interactive manner" (393).

These proposals demonstrate a confluent interest in two areas of thinking that philosophers and literary theorists have been working on for at least the past fifty years, namely, the systematic uncertainty of our ways of knowing, and the importance of interpersonal, that is, subjective understanding, and of course, misunderstanding.[5] The confluence of empirical and humanist interests suggested by these hypotheses encourages us to rethink the interchange among acting bodies, rhetorical forms and emergent meaning. It unsettles, in particular, the implication that the direction of influence is from artwork to audience.

An important beginning was surely J. L. Austin's recognition revealed in Lecture XI of his William James lectures of 1955, that not only warnings and threats, but all speech acts are performative:

> surely to state is every bit as much to perform as, say, to warn or pronounce.... Once we realize that what we have to study is *not* the sentence but the issuing of an utterance in a speech situation, there can hardly be any longer a possibility of not seeing that stating is performing an act.... It is an act to which it is essential to "secure uptake."[6]

Speech consists entirely of illocutionary acts: all speech is action in that all speech has the power to make things happen, and in speech situations, speakers are interested in the results of their actions. These results are what Austin calls the audience's uptake, by which word he has linked his work to the traditional concern of the rhetorician that speech be bent to influence. Austin did not name audiencing as a speech act; in fact, he explicitly excluded the language of poetry and words spoken on the stage.[7] John Searle, in his classification of Austin's illocutionary acts,[8] followed Austin in this, but let us not miss the cue from their connection of rhetoric, speech acts and motor resonance, and that is that agency is involved: a person (mostly—but not always) chooses to be an audience. Novel reading (school assignments aside), or reading a poem in a periodical isn't forced. People take themselves to the theatre and buy a ticket. They come with expectations, and they agree to certain conditions governing their actions. As literary theorist Mary Louise Pratt, with Austin in mind, describes their action, however, it is clear that audiences also agree, to some extent, to refrain from action. They "knowingly and willingly enter a speech situation in which another speaker has unique access to the floor."[9] Giving up the conventions of conversational turn-taking that offer all participants the opportunity to speak, audiences listen, without interrupting, to the speech of actors in dialogue with each other. Pratt supplements Austin with H. Paul Grice's "cooperative principle," according to which everyday language is guided by conventions of context appropriateness, sufficiency and relevance.[10] She argues that the speech act conventions governing the behaviour of audiences when engaging literary texts and public performances are neither fictional nor part of the rhetoric of fiction, but are versions of the "general appropriateness conditions governing speaker/Audience relations in the most familiar and commonplace speech situations ... which is itself defined in relation to the rhetoric of conversation" (115–16).

But the contract they accept, as Pratt makes clear, doesn't require them to give up reciprocity entirely. Audiences assume that what they hear will be worth their attention, their money and their time. And then, in return for the audience's "giving up the floor," as the words of Shakespeare's Prologues and Epilogues acknowledge, the actors (speaking for the author, of course), submit to the audience's judgment. They acknowledge that they are bound to deserve the audience's attention, and often ask explicitly for approval to be expressed by handclapping. The King, speaking as an Epilogue to *All's Well That Ends Well*, acknowledges this explicitly, stepping out of his role as King of France, to speak in propria persona as an actor. He admits to the fiction he has just participated in but also makes clear that the conventions binding him are nonfictional:

> The king's a beggar, now the play is done;
> All is well ended, if this suit be won,
> That you express content; which we will pay,
> With strife to please you, day exceeding day.
> Ours be your patience then, and yours our parts,
> Your gentle hands lend us, and take our hearts.

The essays here describe audiences' kinesic intelligence, that is, their ability to attend to and make meaning from the motor resonances their texts provide to their own attentive bodies. Our authors do not mention, but do apparently assume, Pratt's claim that the actions of audiences of plays and readers of novels agree at least temporarily to sit quietly and suspend the expression of their judgments about the work until the end of the performance. The speech act of audiencing, it is thus acknowledged, includes instructions on when not to act. But experienced close readers, as Terence Cave puts it, even sitting quietly, will "experience an echoic trace of that action in their own body via the automatic activation of their motor neurons."[11] They will, then "successfully mediate motor resonance, even enhance it, while inserting it into the whole network of cultural and conceptual resources that individual humans have at their disposal" (p. xx). Cave describes the rhetorical patterns he studies as "a kinesic stimulus" that "motivate a kinesic engagement in the world."[12]

I can no more than mention here the apparent parallel between this situation and that of the monkeys who first revealed to the experimenters how, what came to be called mirror neurons, fired when the monkeys were observing the actions of the people around them, while their corresponding motor neurons remained inactive.[13] So just how does this "engagement" work? How does "uptake" happen? How does the concept of a "stimulus" play out in a situation in which audiences conventionally remain quiet, either reading in an armchair, or sitting in a theatre?

And once we're talking about the links between rhetorical figures and what is happening, unseen, in the minds and bodies of audiences, we are in shouting distance of the cognitive hypotheses of Theory of Mind (ToM). Lisa Zunshine was the first to point to a distinction novelists depend on between (on the one hand) the human evolved and automatic hunger that prompts our continuous searches for information about other people, and (on the other), our success in actually learning what we would like to and what we need to know about others. We cannot, apparently, turn off our evolved ToM, that is, the automatic attempt to read the faces, postures and actions of others as indications of their internal states of mind that begins at birth.[14] Kinesic awareness, dependent, of course, on vision, and enhanced by other sense modalities, is the default way people engage with the material stuff in their social environments and with its representations in all media. We are not, however, promised success, and we do indeed often misunderstand the bodily signs we survey.[15] But no matter how often we make mistakes, misinterpret others, we can't help but keep trying, and what we are trying to do, it seems, is guess what action of our own is going to be necessary and appropriate most immediately. Cognitive thinking in developmental psychology, neurobiology and neurophysiology is now producing descriptions of our minds' work as not only active and interactive, but actually predictive.

As Clark describes "brains like ours," the main business of the brains within our bodies is to produce probabilistic predictions ahead of what is happening in the always busy and buzzing world, and to adjust our movements so as to fit them as closely as possible to our body's needs. Our brains are:

> predictive agents, constantly trying to guess at the structure and shape of the incoming sensory array. Such brains are incessantly pro-active, restlessly seeking to generate the sensory data for themselves using the incoming signal (in a surprising inversion of much traditional wisdom) mostly as a means of checking and correcting their best top-down guessing.[16]

In trying to decide which information is sufficiently new and therefore worth attending to, we turn our heads and move our bodies to hear and to focus or refocus more efficiently. Clark points out how we act to position ourselves better to understand, to correct for discomfort and avoid noxious situations, "causing bodily movements that selectively harvest new sensory stimulations."[17] We reach out our hands to explore, or to defend ourselves, not only learning but changing the world to make it easier for us to learn from and easier to live in. Our bodies' action possibilities are affordances in the ongoing effort to secure optimal understanding in the current, but always unstable environment. It is by its own needs, agency and movement that a human body develops and maintains a relationship with itself and with the world.

An additional level of complexity is added when we turn our attempts at mind-reading to the speech acts of fictional characters, searching for evidence of their unseen beliefs and intentions. What we see of them, of course, is delivered through the words—as Zunshine calls them—"flimsy verbal constructions,"[18] on which we turn the same cognitive skills we use daily. The evocation of visual images in words, from the pen of skilled writers, as in paintings and photography, takes advantage of gaps between kinaesthetic and visual information so as to pull audiences into surprising and interesting complexities.[19] Experienced readers of fiction however have additional ways of making meaning from ink on paper, and they enjoy imagined embodiment in proportion to their experience with the generic contracts of fiction.[20] For example, we take pleasure in the discovery of gaps between the expected results of our ToM searches and what the narrative itself uncovers in time, because we predict an expected resolution. We wouldn't be able to enjoy, as many clearly do, tragic, grotesque, even horrifying representations, if we weren't able to suppress what might be motor responses, and instead of acting, imagine ourselves as positioned in a corner as an observer. Experienced audiences distinguish fictional kinaesthetic situations on stage or on the page from their own, although, as Cave says, they may certainly feel and take pleasure in kinesic echoes.

Differently in different genres, times and places, we learn to be more or less aware of the presence and the interventions of the artist, and thus of the obliquity with which we meet fictional minds. The more immersed we are in the fiction, the more the artist's agency recedes, though always manipulating our experience, deepening or attenuating the resonance with the pain or pleasure of the fictional bodies that the audience has (don't forget) actively sought. One of the most important ways we situate an appropriate level of comfort and interest in regard to a work of art is by making a judgment about its genre. In general, comedy and satire distance our bodies from fictional displays of pain, while tragedy moves us closer in.

If, however, even in face-to-face interactions with intimates we can't assume that we can make accurate inferences from their speech acts or reliably read the postures, gestures and facial expressions of others, how much greater must our scepticism be when we are dealing with fictions that we know are regularly and deliberately built out of the complexities of conflicting and unequally reliable sources of information? The kinesic evidence in stories and pictures always allows more than one interpretation and although, in principle, this is not different from the ambiguity of evidence we seek to interpret about the people in the world around us, we know that artists invest heavily in the structural potential of these conflicts if for no other reason than that they are more interesting than the concord we reasonably hope for in daily life.

Suzanne Keen, a serious and thoughtful student of the workings of empathy in fiction, warns against the assumption that empathy, immersive reading, simulation and perspective taking with fictional characters are the same, even though much earlier criticism conflates them all under the heading of identifying with characters. Having argued that "the contract of fictionality offers a no-strings-attached opportunity for emotional transactions of great intensity,"[21] she asks us to notice that the automatic embodied empathy we probably can't help feeling, need not turn into sympathy. For example Mary Crane's essay in this volume suggests that images of stifling confinement prompt an uncomfortable (and therefore repressed) identification with the Macbeths. Indeed surely the contract of fiction allows us to hate a character that we feel we understand very well. An aesthetic engagement might be hostile—might be sadistic, or Machiavellian, enjoyable precisely because the fictionality of the situation keeps us aware that we are not that suffering character, and thus can hate or enjoy a character's punishment without consequences.

We may also enjoy the freedom provided to the protagonists of some genres to speak without the restrictions daily polite conversation can impose. Stanley Cavell recognizes what would be well described as a second-person perspective in his extension of Austin's work on illocutionary acts to opera libretti. He cites the outburst by Dona Elvira to Don Giovanni in Mozart's opera: "Monster, felon, deceiver!" And he labels it a "passionate perlocutionary utterance."[22] When a passionate utterance is directed at you, he argues, it "demands" that you respond; you must recognize your involvement, your responsibility. Your response, for Cavell, acknowledges your responsibility to the person you are addressing. Passionate perlocutionary speech acts are "not meant (merely, only, primarily) to inform," although they may do that. A passionate utterance is, rather, "designed to have consequential effects on the feelings, thoughts, and actions of others to which my proposals must be responsive" (277). While in illocutionary acts, it is "the 'I' who is doing the action … in perlocutionary acts, the 'you' comes essentially into the picture" (180). Passionate utterances (in words or images) demand an active response to their unconventional displays of misbehaviour, bias and emotion. They testify to imbalances of power, reveal conflicting goals. Some make clear understandings that have been implicit, but hitherto unacknowledged, even unrecognized. They demand action. An estimable work of art is likely to be unconventional in a similar way, and to demand a response from whoever has agreed to be an audience, sometimes by making them uncomfortable in their seats.[23]

Dominique Brancher's essay suggests another way in which an audience can be pulled by kinesic resonances—in her example, by touch—into a fictional engagement without empathizing with any of the characters, in an erotically charged text. That images do this needs no argument. Her essay reminded me of the statue of the hermaphrodite in the Louvre. The statue is called the Sleeping Hermaphroditus, its posture twisted into what art historians call *contrapposto* (Fig. 12.1).

But the figure is not clearly sleeping, though possibly dreaming. The eyes are closed, but the raised left foot suggests that the skilled sculptor has added a further irony to the primary pathos. The temporary release granted by sleep from the struggles of daily life—and how much more so for a body punished by the gods with two sexes—is denied. The body is not at ease, but has forced itself into the contrapposto position, suggesting

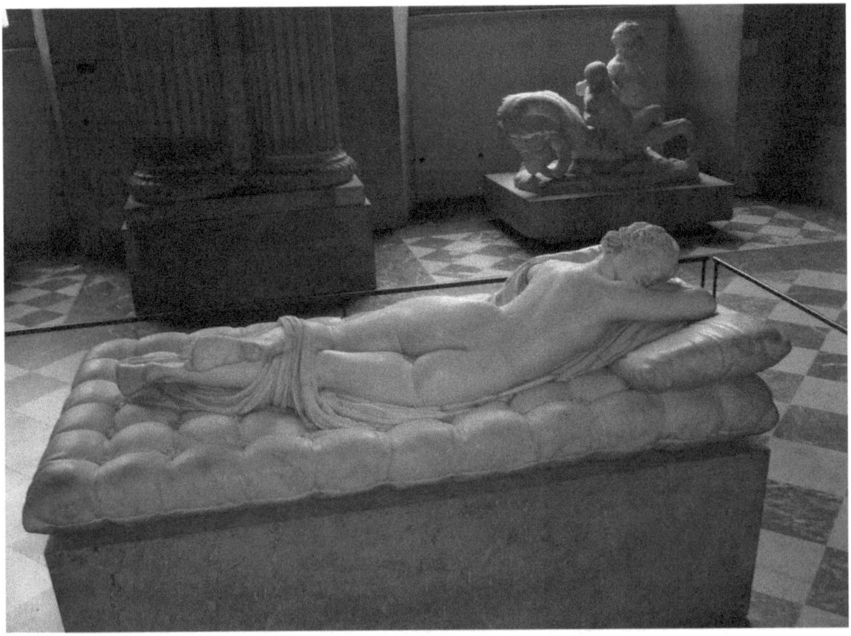

Fig. 12.1 *The Sleeping Hermaphroditus*, a Roman copy of a Greek 2nd c. statue, on a mattress sculpted by Bernini, 1620. Louvre, Paris

the two competing possibilities side by side. The art historian, David Summers, assuming the connections between kinesic resonance and symbolic form, as we have, describes *contrapposto* as the visual equivalent of the rhetorical device of *antithesis*. The posture, Summers says, wherever it is used, has the effect of an argument without a predictable outcome.[24] We know what we know about the correlates of others' postures because they speak to our own proprioception, though that speech can be ambiguous, as our intermittent success in detecting other's states of mind, and as the statue of the Hermaphrodite makes clear. The double genitals are more problematic, however, and may prevent empathy, even while evoking sympathy.[25] The statue thus asks an unconventional, emotional and embodied response: a response from *you*.

The theory needed to describe this kinesic intelligence will surely benefit from the further elaborations of a second-person perspective, such as suggested by Austin, Pratt, Zunshine, Keen, Cavell and Schilbach according to which we are not just viewers, but audience-participants who have accepted a degree of responsibility. The audiences' embodied alignment (or lack thereof) with fictional protagonists makes it impossible to consider them passive observers; the encounter might even be considered a site of conflict. It seems worthwhile to take up Cavell's challenge to recognize responsibility, to work out the contradictions, or foresee the impossibility of so doing.

In closing, I would like to look at a couple of pictures that can give us an idea of the second-person demands made on audiences by kinesic information, and point, as well, to the gradience of those demands. The neuroimaging studies performed and surveyed by Schilbach et al. have to rely on software that measures interest by tracking visual attention, gaze movement and fixation in response to "virtual characters" presented to subjects immobilized in an MRI machine.[26] We can do better, however. Look, for example, at this Italian baroque representation said to represent a scene from the apocryphal story of Susanna and the Elders (Fig. 12.2).[27]

Chiari has painted Susanna in an extremely unhappy and uncomfortable position. Susanna, in both of the Greek sources, is the virtuous wife threatened by two lascivious old men. Her face expresses her distress at being discovered in the private activity of a bath, but more revealing of her pain is her twisted body, as she tries to push away one of the intruders with her right arm which, at that angle could have little force. She tries simultaneously to pull a cover over her body with her left arm, but is successful at neither. Although she wishes not to be seen, the painter's goal is that she indeed be seen; that her desirability, and also their lustful abuse, be revealed.[28] Her contrapposto produces this conflict, a double direction of inference. Her body's torsion suggests not only what has already happened—she has become aware of their aggression. But because she cannot maintain this twisted position for long, something else has to happen, which we are left to infer. The audience may be inclined to sympathy with the woman, who looks up with a pleading dismay. But a second-person perspective is also open: because of what you as audience see, you are accused, with the elders, as an intruder, an offender. The painter has put the viewer in a position demanding a physical response: you are addressed and asked to turn away. So drop the pretence of the story frame of Susanna—you, assumed to be a male viewer, are asked to stop staring, stop enjoying the woman's discomfort—even the picture of a woman's discomfort: move away!

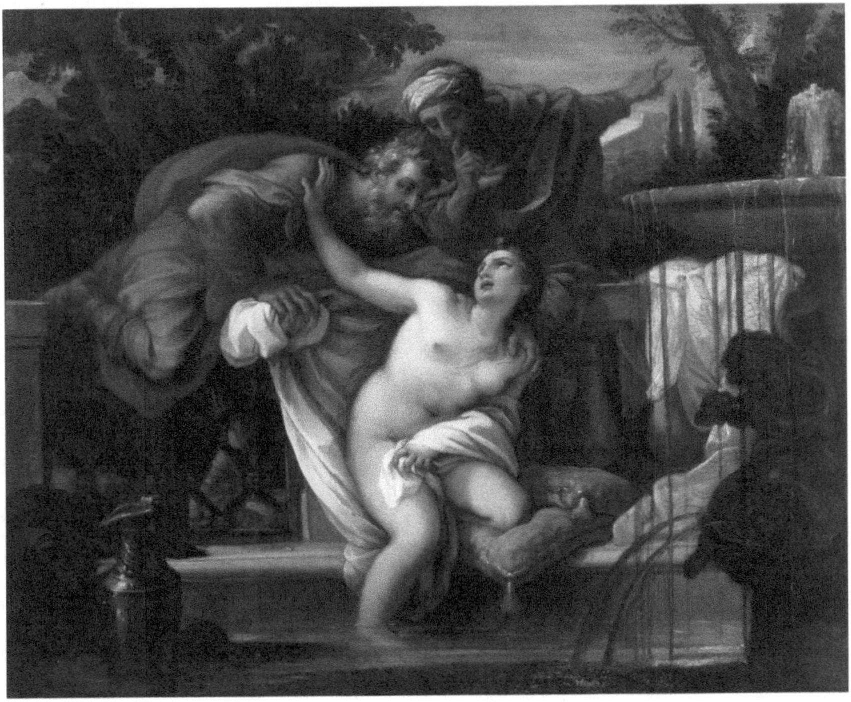

Fig. 12.2 Giuseppe Bartolomeo Chiari, *Susanna and the Elders*, Walters Art Museum, Baltimore, Maryland

In Caravaggio's *Doubting Thomas* many people feel the abuse of Thomas's probing finger, and may be further discomfited by noticing the corresponding erotic slit in the offender's garment (Fig. 12.3).

Caravaggio positions the three apostles leaning in toward Jesus, but the viewer of the painting—it's a large one—may recoil from it, lean backward in disgust.[29] The kinesic reaction here is additionally complicated because viewers won't recognize what is happening, and how they are being personally addressed, unless they belong to the community that knows the story. Post-Tridentine religious history painting, like the best news photography today, clearly intended to evoke strong emotions and produce active response in audiences. The photojournalist, like the painter of religious narratives, addresses a community assumed to be "second person": prima facie involved and ready to respond.

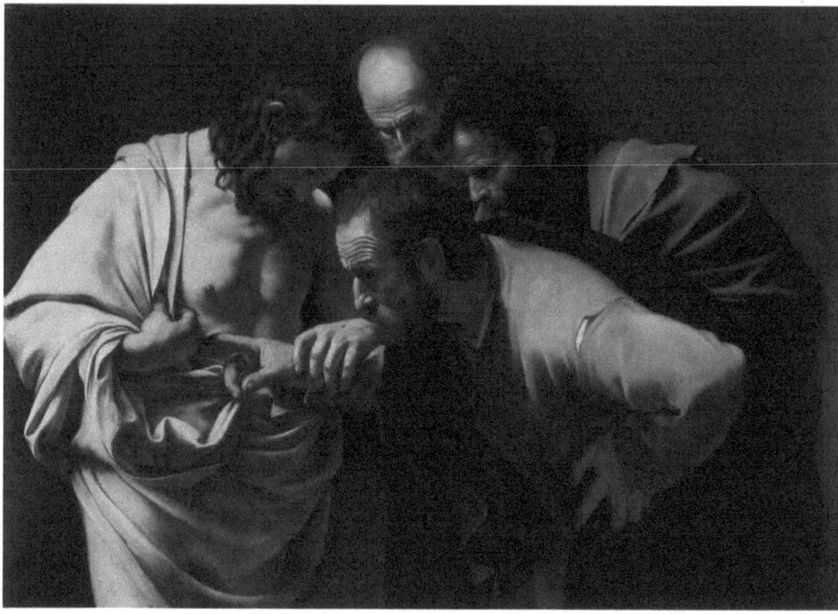

Fig. 12.3 Caravaggio, *Doubting Thomas* (1602–1603), Sanssouci, Potsdam

Successful artists have always known that multiplying sensory information adds complexity to our experience by surprising their audiences with multiple perspectives. Scholarly attention to the impact of the kinaesthetic communications of motor imagery, generalizing from the recognitions of ToM, and taking into account our evolved hunger for information about the people around us, allow us to infer plot possibilities by hypothesizing future actions or rethinking the implications of past movements.[30] The term intake as used by psychologists describing a body's reception of information from the world, likely specifies the same aspect of the action that Austin called uptake, and, as Clark describes it, the mind decides which specific bits of outside stuff are worth importing, engaging and processing, based on previous experience.

> The picture that here emerges is one of neural encodings that are *fundamentally* in the business of action control. Such encodings represent how the world is in ways that are entwined, at multiple levels, with information about how to act upon the world."[31]

Clark paraphrases, here, the "affordance competition hypothesis" of neurologist Paul Cisek who puts it this way it on his website:

> the brain is continuously using sensory information to specify potential actions available in the world ("affordances") while at the same time collecting cues for selecting which one is most appropriate at a given moment.[32]

Literary texts, like all imaginative creations, are affordances in this sense. Given the substantial evidence for the reuse of the same neural paths that see or act for recreating those scenes or actions imaginatively, there is no reason to exclude the simulations that our interactions with imaginative texts encourage from this general account of cognition. Works of the imagination, on this view, are prompts, chosen for attentive elaboration as needed by current audiences in their contexts. The interaction undertaken, then, the second-person perspective, keeps it in motion. Vittorio Gallese has also argued for a second-person perspective in describing social interaction. "The motor aspects of the bodily self," he says, "provide the means to integrate self-related multimodal sensory information about the body and the world it interacts with."[33] And Schilbach:

> Knowing others is [not] limited to perceiving them. We argue for an approach to social knowing based on interaction and emotional engagements between people, rather than mere observation. This second-person approach has already begun to prove productive within developmental and social psychology and points toward the importance of experiencing and interacting with others as our primary ways of knowing them.[34]

Notes

1. Chaim Perelman and L. Olbrechts-Tyteca, *The New Rhetoric: A Treatise on Argumentation* (Notre Dame: Notre Dame University Press, 1969).
2. See David Duff, "Melodies of Mind: Poetic Forms as Cognitive Structures," in *Cognition, Literature, and History*, ed. Mark J. Bruhn and Donald R. Wehrs (New York: Routledge, 2014), 17–38, for an account of how rhetorical figures have been linked, starting with Longinus, and through eighteenth-century theories of the sublime, to bodily knowledge such as has been called "hot cognition" by psychologist Herbert Simon.
3. Oxford: Oxford University Press, 2016.

4. Schilbach et al., “Toward a second-person neuroscience,” *Behavioral and Brain Sciences* 36 (2013): 393–414, https://doi.org/10.1017/S0140525X12000660.
5. On misunderstanding, see Ellen Spolsky, *The Contracts of Fiction: Cognition, Culture, Community* (New York: Oxford University Press, 2015), 130–154.
6. *How to Do Things with Words* (Oxford: Oxford University Press, 1962), 134, 139.
7. For a discussion of this odd mistake of Austin’s, see Spolsky, *The Contracts of Fiction*, 137–38, 239.
8. John Searle, “A Classification of Illocutionary Acts,” *Language in Society* 5 (1976): 1–23.
9. *Toward a Speech Act Theory of Literary Discourse* (Bloomington, IN: Indiana University Press, 1977), 114.
10. H. Paul Grice, “Logic and Conversation,” in *Syntax and Semantics, vol. 3: Speech Acts*, ed. Peter Cole and Jerry Morgan (New York: Academic Press, 1975).
11. In this volume, p. x.
12. *Thinking with Literature: Towards a Cognitive Criticism* (Oxford: Oxford University Press, 2016), 83.
13. An early report was G. Rizzolatti et al., “Premotor Cortex and the Recognition of Motor Actions,” *Cognitive Brain Research* 3 (1996): 131–41. Hundreds of studies have followed, including a subset discussing the relevance to literary theory and criticism, for which see Lisa Zunshine, “Lying Bodies of the Enlightenment: Theory of Mind and Cultural Historicism,” in *Introduction to Cognitive Cultural Studies*, ed. Lisa Zunshine (Baltimore, MD: The Johns Hopkins University Press, 2010), 115–33.
14. Lisa Zunshine, *Why We Read Fiction: Theory of Mind and the Novel* (Columbus: The Ohio State University Press, 2006), 6ff; Zunshine, “Lying Bodies.”
15. Zunshine, *Why We Read Fiction*, 13.
16. *Surfing Uncertainty*, 3.
17. *Surfing Uncertainty*, 7.
18. *Why We Read Fiction*, 10.
19. See Spolsky, *Gaps in Nature: Literary Interpretation and the Modular Mind* (Albany: SUNY UP, 1993).
20. Spolsky, *The Contracts of Fiction*.
21. *Empathy and the Novel* (Oxford: Oxford University Press, 2007), 168. See also Keen’s “Pivoting Toward Empiricism,” *Narrative* 24 (2016).
22. Stanley Cavell, “Performative and Passionate Utterance,” in *Philosophy the Day after Tomorrow* (Cambridge, MA: Harvard University Press, 2005), 155–91.

23. See Spolsky, "An Embodied View of Misunderstanding in *Macbeth*," *Poetics Today* 32 (2011): 489–520, for more on passionate performances and responsibility.
24. "Contrapposto: Style and Meaning in Renaissance Art," *The Art Bulletin* 59 (1977): 347.
25. You might want to look at the collection of pictures of the statue in Google Images where you can see it from several other angles than the one shown here.
26. "Toward a second-person neuroscience."
27. The scene in which the elders surprise the naked young wife in her bath, although repeatedly painted by European painters, does not occur in the text. See Ellen Spolsky, *Satisfying Skepticism: Embodied Knowledge in the Early Modern World* (Aldershot: Ashgate, 2001) for a fuller discussion of this story of Susanna, and of several Doubting Thomas pictures as well.
28. The sculptor of the Louvre Hermaphrodite similarly benefits from presenting the subject as failing to conceal what the audience is of course interested in.
29. Rembrandt's "Doubting Thomas" (see it on Google Images), in Moscow, has Thomas leaning back and away from what he sees.
30. On interpreting pictured postures as predictive, see Spolsky, "Elaborated Knowledge: Reading Kinesis in Pictures," *Poetics Today* 17 (1996): 162.
31. *Surfing Uncertainty*, 181.
32. http://www.cisek.org/pavel
33. "Bodily selves in relation: embodied simulation as second-person perspective on intersubjectivity," *Philosophical Transactions of the Royal Society B*, 369 (2014). https://doi.org/10.1098/rstb.2013.0177.
34. Schilbach et al., "Toward a second-person neuroscience," 3.

Bibliography

Austin, J. L. *How to Do Things with Words.* Oxford: Oxford University Press, 1962.

Cave, Terence. *Thinking with Literature: Towards a Cognitive Criticism.* Oxford: Oxford University Press, 2016.

Cavell, Stanley. Performative and Passionate Utterance. In *Philosophy the Day After Tomorrow*, 155–91. Cambridge, MA: Harvard University Press, 2005.

Cisek, Paul. 2010. http://www.cisek.org/pavel

Clark, Andy. *Surfing Uncertainty: Prediction, Action, and the Embodied Mind.* Oxford: Oxford University Press, 2016.

Duff, David. Melodies of Mind: Poetic Forms as Cognitive Structures. In *Cognition, Literature, and History*, ed. Mark J. Bruhn and Donald R. Wehrs, 17–38. New York: Routledge, 2014.

Gallese, Vittorio. Bodily Selves in Relation: Embodied Simulation as Second-Person Perspective on Intersubjectivity. *Philosophical Transactions of the Royal Society B*, 369 (2014). https://doi.org/10.1098/rstb.2013.0177.

Grice, H. Paul. Logic and Conversation. In *Syntax and Semantics, vol. 3: Speech Acts*, ed. Peter Cole and Jerry Morgan, 41–58. New York: Academic Press, 1975.

Keen, Suzanne. *Empathy and the Novel.* Oxford: Oxford University Press, 2007.

———. Pivoting Toward Empiricism. *Narrative* 24 (2016).

Perelman, Chaim, and L. Olbrechts-Tyteca. *The New Rhetoric: A Treatise on Argumentation.* Notre Dame: Notre Dame University Press, 1969.

Pratt, Mary Louise. *Toward a Speech Act Theory of Literary Discourse.* Bloomington, IN: Indiana University Press, 1977.

Rizzolatti, G., L. Fadiga, V. Gallese, and L. Fogassi. Premotor Cortex and the Recognition of Motor Actions. *Cognitive Brain Research* 3 (1996): 131–41.

Schilbach, Leonhard, Bert Timmermans, Vasudevi Reddy, Alan Costall, Gary Bente, Tobias Schlicht, and Kai Vogeley. Toward a Second-Person Neuroscience. *Behavioral and Brain Sciences* 36 (2013): 393–414. https://doi.org/10.1017/S0140525X12000660.

Searle, John. A Classification of Illocutionary Acts. *Language in Society* 5 (1976): 1–23.

Spolsky, Ellen. *Gaps in Nature: Literary Interpretation and the Modular Mind.* Albany: SUNY UP, 1993.

———. Elaborated Knowledge: Reading Kinesis in Pictures. *Poetics Today* 17 (1996): 157–80.

———. *Satisfying Skepticism: Embodied Knowledge in the Early Modern World.* Aldershot: Ashgate, 2001.

———. An Embodied View of Misunderstanding in *Macbeth. Poetics Today* 32 (2011): 489–520.

———. *The Contracts of Fiction: Cognition, Culture, Community.* New York: Oxford University Press, 2015.

Summers, David. Contrapposto: Style and Meaning in Renaissance Art. *The Art Bulletin* 59 (1977): 336–61.

Zunshine, Lisa. *Why We Read Fiction: Theory of Mind and the Novel.* Columbus: The Ohio State University Press, 2006.

———. Lying Bodies of the Enlightenment: Theory of Mind and Cultural Historicism. In *Introduction to Cognitive Cultural Studies*, edited by Lisa Zunshine, 115–33. Baltimore, MD: The Johns Hopkins University Press, 2010.

Index[1]

[1] Note: Page numbers followed by "n" refer to notes.

K. Banks, T. Chesters (eds.), *Movement in Renaissance Literature*, Cognitive Studies in Literature and Performance,
https://doi.org/10.1007/978-3-319-69200-5

T

Kolibri 360 GmbH
Ferdinand-Jühlke-Straße 7
99095 Erfurt, Deutschland
produktsicherheit@kolibri360.de